Take your brick walls
lay them flat and make
them stepping stones.

Yvonne L. Williams

Tested Faith

The Power of Mind Over Cancer

by
Yvonne L. Williams

Copyright © 2000 by Yvonne L. Williams

Robert D. Reed Publishers

750 LaPlaya, Suite 647
San Francisco, CA 94121
Phone: 650-994-6570 • Fax: -6579
E-mail: 4bobreed@msn.com
http://www.rdrpublishers.com

Typesetter: **Barbara Kruger**
Editor: **Colin Ingram**
Cover design: **Irene Taylor, it grafx**
Artwork: **Dave Ali, Trinidad, W.I.**

ISBN 1-885003-67-6

Library of Congress Catalog Card Number 00-105267

Manufactured, typeset and printed in the United States of America

Dedicated to

My beloved sister, Leah Y. Sun-Seargent, RN,CNM
and
The nurses at Baystate Medical Center
Springfield, Massachusetts

I would not exchange the sorrows of my heart
for the joys of the multitude. And I would
not have the tears that sadness makes to flow
from my every part turn into laughter. I
would that my life remain a tear and a smile.

Kahill Gibran

Acknowledgments

American Cancer Society
Massachusetts Division, Inc.
Jacqueline Baez, MD
Julia Donovan, MD
Kevin T. Hinchey, MD
Paul S. Farkas, MD
Ronald Kanagaki, MD
Robert J. Kasper, MD, F.A.C.S.
Persio Ballista, MD
Enid V. Blaylock, Ph.D.
Rochelle Curtis, SEER Group
National Institutes of Health, Bethesda, Maryland
Ann MacMillan, Massachusetts Cancer Registry, Boston, MA

Special Thanks To:
William, Phyllis, my mother, Robert, Danielle, Gail, Lincoln, Sandy, Eric, Charlene, Agnes, Vickie, Libby, Carol and all my other friends and family who have supported me, and made this book possible.

Thanks, you are wonderful!
Dave Ali, Enid Blaylock, Ph.D, Sandra Falconer, Laura Edwards, Carla Riccio, David Hiatt, Selwyn Cudjoe, Ph.D., Elaine Anderson, Ed.D., Deb Axtel, Jewel Pookram, M.D., Ph.D.

Foreword
by Enid V. Blaylock, Ph.D.

Yvonne L. Williams, the author of this inspiring book, is a very unusual wife and mother whose optimistic world-view has endeared her to family, friends and strangers alike. She radiates life—cheerfulness, joy and high spirits. And, above all, she is ready and willing to help others.

Her willingness to share was the primary motive for writing Tested Faith, a book that is likely to help not only cancer sufferers garner the strength and courage to fight for their lives but it provides insight into the psychological battle one goes through in coping with cancer.

The diagnosis of cancer is a devastating experience that invokes depressing thoughts. I was in such a state, having recently been diagnosed with cancer, when I received a telephone call from the author, my niece. She said, "Aunt E, you must decide that you want to live. Your mind and will have power over your body. You can will yourself to live. Set a goal," she said. "'As a man thinketh in his heart, so is he.' Tell yourself you want to see your grandchildren grow up and finish college."

Although my prognosis was dismal, her strong conviction and positive outlook dispelled my feeling of resignation, and I became a cancer survivor going on several years. I have no doubt that she can do the same for others through her writing. A particularly useful aspect of the knowledge she imparts relates to such activities as exercise, diet, self-love, and avoidance of prolonged negative stress and maintenance of a positive attitude.

Her zest for life, determination and unshakable faith in God comes through loud and clear. These positive forces will influence readers in ways that lead to a new lease on life, a new way of thinking about mind/body relationship and a high level of confidence in the degree of control one has over one's destiny.

Contents

Introduction

Over the course of years I have interviewed over 500 persons who have had cancer or some other potentially fatal disease. The common thread running throughout all is a tendency towards despair—the difficulty in holding on to hope. There are few things in life that push one into great despair as being told that one has cancer or any catastrophic illness. All sense of rational thinking is lost as negative emotions rise within one's innermost being and take control of the psyche. A brief flame of disbelief lights but is quickly snuffed out as the reality of the doctor's words begins to sink in.

How clearly I remember the initial difficulty in holding onto faith, "The substance of things hoped for, the evidence of things not seen," in hopes that eventually the evidence will be seen. Exercising explicit belief that I could be healed and was going to live in the face of three cancers was one of life's greatest challenges for me. To sustain and implement mountain-moving faith is near impossible. Making the mental and environmental changes that are necessary to support that type of faith is a challenge within itself. The daily perseverance that supports the mental and environmental changes are unyielding. The minute-by-minute, negative psychological warfare that goes on within one's head in the face of such a challenge is inconceivable.

When I was dying from cancer, I had to hold onto something more tangible than the physicians' prognosis or the effects of innovative treatments. I could not hold onto someone else's faith, or someone's religious beliefs and prayers. In my heart, I believed without a doubt that if I could win the head game, I could beat cancer. Therefore, I had to take hold of my faith and keep it shielded, impervious to thoughts that could weaken my right to hope and my will to persevere.

Eleven years have passed since I engaged in the struggle to beat cancer. Stirring up my memories, I remembered April 17, 1989, the day I found that I was afflicted with a cancer. On May 17 of that year I was operated on for three primary cancers (cancer that had not spread):

ovarian (both ovaries), colon and endometrial. My struggle to live, I must tell you, was lonely and very difficult at first. The pain, inner shame and outward scourge that accompany cancer forced me to adopt clandestine behaviors. It was not until I decided I wanted to live and anchored myself firmly in God, who gave me hope in order for me to exercise my mustard seed faith, and only when my mind was fully renewed, that the healing process started.

Tested Faith is a unique testament that resulted from much prayer and meditation, and a desire to share my life-changing experience with others. My challenge with three primary cancers was not a journey of death, but rather a pathway to physical, spiritual, emotional and mental growth—a wake-up call for me to engage life and find my purpose for being. The body's disease is a drastic call for change, for internal realignment and harmony.

Conceived as a catalyst to initiate change and a message of inspiration and hope to all, Tested Faith candidly chronicles my painful self-analysis that forced me to take full ownership for my behaviors; behaviors that I believe contributed to my illness. It narrates my psychological difficulties and details my fears; but most importantly, it documents my triumph over ego and the realignment of my body.

I do not consider myself a cancer survivor, but a victor over cancer. I refused to be submissive to cancer and let it dictate my destiny and my mental prowess. I have refused to keep the cancer connectivity and look at myself as just a survivor. It is because of my boldness, not humility; my faith, not fear; my passion, not pity, that there are no permanent scars from my experience except for the marks left by the surgeon's scalpel. There are no clouds of reoccurrence or possible reoccurrence hanging over my head, nor does a list of cancer survival strategies accompany me during my daily activities. My hopes for winning the insatiable battle with cancer was never predicated on miracle drugs, surgery or isolation and treatment of mutated genes. From early on I realized that I was the caretaker of my body and victory lay within me, within my mind. Therefore, geared with understanding, the renewal of my mind, faith in God and an excellent medical team, I was able to be victorious over a relentless competitor.

More than eight million Americans, including myself, who have a history of cancer are alive today. But sad to say, there are approximately 1,252,000 new cancer cases per year. However, few will survive three or more primary cancers. The tide must be slowed!

As a victor, I find it important to let others know how factors such as prolonged internalization of negative stress, anger, unhappiness, hate, both of others and self and resentment are poisons. The biochemical reactions that negative stress produces break down the immune system and leave us susceptible to catastrophic illness. In addition, refusing to be all that we can be causes internal conflict (dis-ease) and puts us at risk of being catastrophically ill.

Tested Faith will help the public understand that our bodies are temples and that we, and only we, are keepers of those delicate temples. No one can force us to take care of ourselves, nor will us to live. Neither can the doctors medicate us to life-long health. Loving ourselves and taking care of our bodies is a conscious and singular choice each one of us has to make.

I am convinced above all else that loving myself, my faith in God, the renewing of my mind and my willingness to make permanent changes in my environment are the four most important factors that allowed me to achieve full and lasting recovery from cancer.

I have learned during the years to "Take my brick walls, lay them flat and make them stepping stones."

1

The Disturbing Telephone Call

The Lord takes us into troubled waters,
Not to drown us, but to cleanse us.
                                    Author Unknown

On April 17, 1989—a day never to be forgotten—my dress was casual because it was going to be a long day auditing inventory at the plant. What a needed release from the regimens and formality of my usual routine.

As it turned out, the rhythm of the day was exciting as I traveled from area to area to meet people and review the auditing progress. But as the morning rolled on, fatigue took hold of me and I began to feel unusually exhausted. The fact that April was always a strenuous time of the year and I was working long hours, made the tired feeling acceptable. It was not out of the ordinary. However, the stairs that I had walked up and down with ease for the last seven years became very difficult to climb. Although obviously weak in the knees, I discarded the thought that I might be ill and continued with my responsibilities. Exhaustion was not unfamiliar to me, but matters were compounded when sporadic dizzy spells seized me and swayed my body, forcing me to rest for a while. In spite of these symptoms, for some unknown reason I continued to push myself to finish the tasks at hand. My body was not in agreement with my wishes. It decisively expressed the need to sit and rest. In response to its commands, I retreated to my office. Looking back, I must confess that in my life there was this unfathomable behavior that constantly pushed me to persist in spite of my physical condition. Therefore, as I retreated to my office, I was more interested in getting my work done than resting, and for that reason, I decided, I would kick off my shoes, elevate my legs and review my morning's correspondence.

Stealing a few seconds to look outside before getting down to business, I found newness to the area. This surprised me. Meditatively, I realized that recently I had not taken time from my daily activities to just sit and stare. My busy schedule prevented me from incorporating such leisure activities into my daily workload. The few seconds turned into minutes. Adding to my surprise, a car wash that was under construction was almost completed. I marveled at the speed with which the construction was proceeding.

Seizing that moment of escape, my eyes traveled to the clear, blue sky. The sun was bright, giving a false sense of summer's warmth. The few fleecy clouds in the sky moved slowly, intermingling with thin symmetrical cloud-like lines that looked like airplane contrails. The air, I remembered, was crisp and clean when I walked from my car to the plant. The night's dark clouds were gone. The relentless outpouring of early morning showers cleansed the atmosphere of impurities. It was as if nature was participating in its own spring-cleaning.

Spring in New England is always beautiful, I thought. A refreshing reprise after winter's cold. It dawned on me that spring was on its way. Soon I would be planting flowers in my own garden. And there in that hiatus between winter and spring I thought of Alice Walker's mother preparing her garden and how she luxuriated in the effulgence of spring in the expression of her own artistic impulse. A Caribbean sunrise seemed to be on the horizon.

This peaceful escapade, however, did not last very long as the ringing of my telephone interrupted it. Momentarily, I thought of not responding and continuing to savor the peace of this beautiful April day. The ringing persisted. Reluctantly, I answered it.

Anna, a manager who worked for me, was on the line. Sounding relieved, she said: "I was just about to hang up. I have looked everywhere for you. Your office was the last place I expected to find you." Sharing my condition with her, I ended casually, "I am probably anemic and need to take iron supplements." That was all I needed to feel better.

Yet at the end of our conversation, a troubling silence fell between us. Exhaling loudly as if she had been holding her breath, Anna breathlessly informed me that someone at the doctor's office had called and requested that I return the call as soon as possible.

"The person said that it is important that you return the call today. I will get back with you, to see if you placed that call," she said, aware of my busy work schedule.

Surprised, I asked, "Which doctor?"

"Your gynecologist, Dr. Baez."

"Dr. Baez?"

The pleasant interlude was completely swept away by Anna's message. Bristling with sudden concern, my body went tense. What does this call mean? Suddenly, it seemed as if my heart had dropped and was gripped by an inexplicable fear. The initial moment of silence between us was overtaken by an unspoken fear and understanding about the doctor's request that I return her call ASAP. Anna broke the silence by giving me Dr. Baez's number while offering her support.

"I'll call a little later." Although I tried to sound light-hearted, the strain in my voice was obvious.

"Okay, I will check with you after lunch," Anna replied in a motherly voice. In spite of her maternal kindness, this exchange between Anna and me was fraught with a peculiar type of uneasiness. Sensing that something might be dreadfully wrong I began to fight back tears of anxiety. Unwarranted or not, skepticism set in like gangrene and instantly my mind began an active search for answers. Nothing else mattered as I tried to decipher why this disturbing call should arrive when it did. In no time, my legs gained strength as I paced the office floor, walking, worrying. I must have walked a mile, and wore a hole in my heart with worry.

It was my custom to file away unpleasant thoughts until I was prepared to deal with them, and I did this with the doctor's call. Unconsciously, I think, I tried to discount its importance, postponing the inevitable. Yet inescapably, for three hours, fear lurked in the back of my head as I worried about the message. Unable to bear the suspense any longer, I summoned enough courage and dialed the doctor's number with weak optimism.

"Hello, my name is Yvonne Williams, I am returning Dr. Baez's call." I said with cautious steadiness in my voice.

"Hello, Mrs. Williams, Dr. Baez would like to see you this afternoon. The doctor has 4:00 p.m. open, can you make it?"

My body grew tense and my brittle optimism began to fall apart when I heard the words at the end of the telephone. I tried rescheduling the appointment, thinking that if the appointment could be rescheduled, then the visit was not necessarily important. "My scheduled is booked up this afternoon, what about tomorrow? By the way, what is this visit all about?" I asked nonchalantly, but scared stiff to find out.

"I do not know, but it is important that you keep the appointment."

Shaken by the response, my mind began to play frantic, dubious games with me—wandering, conjecturing, touching and exploring every imaginable illness associated with the uterus. Having cancer had never crossed my mind before, but the call from the doctor now trumped up thoughts of this frightening disease. "God help it not to be cancer," I threw up a prayer in desperation.

Cancer was familiar to me through others I knew who had been afflicted; close friends and relatives. I watched them change from happy outgoing persons, seemingly healthy in every way, to somber, fearful patients burdened by the weight of their illness. Oftentimes, I had tried to help them recognize the healing power of God in spite of their doubts. "Trust in God and do not doubt." Those were the words from my childhood, spoken to my grandfather in his illness. If I had cancer, could I take the same medicine I had often dished out? Could I trust God and not doubt? I discarded the mental discourse. The whole notion was irrelevant.

Yet the persistent concerns remained and I became anxious and nervous. My thoughts scampered back and forth. Vigorously, I shook my head as if this action would throw unwanted thoughts to the bottom and allow me to reinstate a hold over my thoughts and emotions and ignore the possibilities.

In the afternoon, Anna came by my office as she had promised to inquire if I had called the doctor. With arms akimbo, she asked skeptically.

"Did you place that call?"

Anna's arrival cut into my anguish.

"Yes," I answered, my face masqueraded in a smile.

Sick with anxiety, I was tempted to blurt out, "The doctor has to give me bad news that cannot wait," but I resisted all show of uneasiness. Instinctively I felt Anna knew that I was concerned. Women carry these sensitivities within them. It's like a kind of spiritual Geiger counter that tells them when something is wrong, especially when it has to do with another woman. Camouflaging my fear, I told her that the doctor had asked me to visit her that afternoon. She immediately volunteered to take me, reminding me of my ill feeling. Thanking her, I cordially declined her offer. Bad news should be heard alone.

Anna was not easily deterred. She firmly insisted that she would accompany me, giving additional reasons why she thought I needed to have someone with me on this important—and perhaps painful—occasion.

Although Anna had worked for me for couple of years, it was still difficult to share this intimate aspect of my life with her. I was entering the unknown and preferred to explore that territory alone. To accommodate her willingness to help, I told her that if I changed my mind I would let her know. I was not ready to throw off that wall of reserve that had kept me wrapped up within the castle of my Caribbean skin. But then, touched by her kindness, I finally accepted. Perhaps more than I cared to admit, I needed the comforting presence of a friend to see me through this ordeal.

Anna arrived on time to drive me to see Dr. Baez. The drive was silent. Tense with anticipation, I was in a no-talking mood. My palms oozed sweat and my breathing came in short bursts as I sat tensed with fear; I knew that something was dreadfully wrong.

Soon we arrived. The distance to Dr. Baez's office seemed shorter than usual. My heart accelerated its beat as I entered the patients' waiting room, cloaked in trepidation.

The waiting room was alive. Patients kept coming and going. I tried to calm my shattered nerves and remove my mind from the discussion that was going to take place by engaging Anna with busy chatter, while also nervously browsing through People Magazine with trembling fingers. Nothing registered. My eyes were blinded to the contents of the pages. Nervous, I could not settle down and wait. Now and again I glanced at the door that led to the inner offices, hopefully wishing that the nurse would come out, call my name and inform me that my being there was all a big mistake.

Thoughts raced back and forth in my head as I waited to be called. March 27, 1989, Janet King, one of my best friends, insisted that I call Dr. Jacqueline Baez, my gynecologist, to make an appointment to see her. The warning that came from that melodious Jamaican voice was stern but friendly: "Girl, I am tired of you missing your appointments because of unscheduled meetings. One day, you are going to drop dead in one of them. I am going to make an appointment for you and I will take you there personally."

My friend's remarks haunted me as I went over the events of the day.

It was because of Jan's urging that I saw Dr. Baez on April 3, 1989, and underwent a D&C, the cleaning out of the uterus, on April 7, 1989. It was probably the results from the D&C that prompted the call from Dr. Baez. In spite of my anxiety, oh how thankful I was for Jan's insisting that I visit the doctor. I heard the name "Yvonne Williams" called, seemingly a distant echo of a name I knew in the past, uttered in a different manner and in an intonation connected with some gloom. My answer was soft and awkward. It was apparent as I was ushered by the nurse into the doctor's private office—not to the examination room—that something was wrong.

With her ever-present charming and reassuring smile, Dr. Baez welcomed me and offered pleasantries. I was not deceived. Her pensive demeanor and carefully enunciated words began to play on my worst fears. She was honest and precise with the information. But the qualitative contexts of her statements were hard to digest.

Looking demurely and directly into my eyes, she said, "I have received and reviewed the results of your D&C and cancer was found in your endometrial lining."

In response, I threw a terrified glance at the doctor and hoped she did not notice it. The shock was stinging and I stifled my impulse to cry out in response. A chill of silence fell over the room as Dr. Baez's words hung in the air like suspended icicles. It was a moment of truth that forever affected me. It took some time for me to translate what she had said. Stunned, I sat clutching my hands tightly together as this dreaded phenomenon began to unfold. "Oh no! Oh no!" I thought, "My God, how long has this cancer been growing in my body?" I had to know the answer. A lump formed in my throat and I had to clear it before asking.

"How long have I had it?" I was too scared to even mention the word cancer.

"I do not know," she replied as if carefully choosing her words.

"Has the cancer spread to different parts of my body?" I asked, fearing the worst and not wanting to hear the answer.

"The results I have were strictly based on the D&C. I have no additional information. More tests will have to be performed to determine the extent of the disease."

Biting my lips, I shook my head in disbelief. I could not believe that this was happening to me. Gently touching my hand, Dr. Baez asked, "Do you have any questions?"

"Tell me this is a dream, please tell me!" I wanted to cry out. But instead I answered, as my senses became dazed. "No, I have no questions."

"Are you sure?"

"Yes, I'm sure." My throat felt instantly parched from an inward heat. I swallowed to cool it. The unremitting palpitation of my heart beat loudly against my breast as I unsuccessfully tried to relax. It is impossible to describe my true feelings.

Dr. Baez looked at me with sympathetic eyes as she continued; "Yvonne, this is not the end. There are thousands who have been cured of cancer. We have to determine the extent of your cancer, then proceed with the best possible treatment."

Her statements were not registering as my mind raced with calamitous thoughts. Her next question brought me back to the reality of the situation.

"Would you like me to inform your husband?" She offered to assist me in breaking the news to my loved ones.

The strength in me was all gone but my response was strong and certain. "No. No, thank you. I want to tell him."

"Have thine own way, Lord! Have thine own way! Wounded and weary, Help me I pray! Power, all power, surely is thine! Touch me and heal me, Savior divine." Shaken as I was, Mamma's (my grandmother) soothing voice was softly singing in my head.

Dr. Baez's voice was soft and full of warmth. "Are you okay, Yvonne?"

She knew I was not, but I answered "yes," forcing a smile of reassurance.

"Is there anyone else in your family you would like me to speak with?"

"No, no one." I heard my voice in the distance—strangely subdued. "This is the voice of pain," I thought.

And the ritual continued. For a moment my head felt dizzy as I held my breath tightly. Dr. Baez's voice sounded hollow as though she was a distance away from me. But somewhere in the mass of incomprehension I heard the name "Dr. Julia Donovan," a surgeon and oncologist recommended to me. I wanted to cry, but I could not, the tears did not flow. Inside, my heart wept with pain.

If I did not know better, I would attest that the floor moved when I stood up. My knees were weaker as I walked towards the waiting room in a daze. There is no memory of me entering the room or seeing Anna. But I remember that as we left Dr. Baez's office, my worry meter shot up several notches, pumping additional adrenaline, cortisol and endorphin into my body. My jaws clenched automatically and my breathing became short and erratic. My furrowed brow became more pronounced, the muscles on my shoulders tightened and burned, and my heart beat faster. I swallowed several times in order to dislodge the lump that blocked my throat. No matter how I swallowed it did not move. It just stuck there. I was engulfed in stress. Without any conscious will, my body was spontaneously responding to news it did not want to hear.

What had befallen me? What had I done to deserve such a catastrophe? I was at the height of my life. Now my life had catapulted into mass confusion and distress within a few minutes. It was a horrible message at this time of my life. "My God!" was my only prayer.

Though the dice were cast, a small bit of light shone through in all of this darkness. My condition was no longer a question, the medical verdict was in. I had a definable illness, and it was treatable. That I could handle. Sadly, I remembered those gone that preferred not to have their symptoms diagnosed and others who refused to accept their diagnosis, thereby eliminating the possibility for cure. Early detection of any illness increases the chance for cure and survivability.

On that bleak spring afternoon—such news would make any afternoon bleak—the one inexpressive thought that came to my lips was "I am going to beat this! I am going to beat this with the help of God, I am going to beat this!"

2

The Natural Consequence of Neglect

Doth not Wisdom cry?
and Understanding
put forth her voice?
                    Proverbs 8:1

Dispirited and scared, my face could not smile for the pain within my heart. I could not see for the tears that swelled in my eyes. Slowly, dejected and blinded by tears, I walked away from the doctor's office, each step dogged by anguish. By all evidence, I understood that surgery does not cure and only a small percentage of medicine cures infections while most only treat symptoms. I knew that chemotherapy and radiation lend hope; they are not cancer cures.

The thought of having cancer and the possible treatments began to play havoc with my fears and my thoughts vacillated between hope and despair. One moment I thought it was the end, the next moment I was hopeful that I would beat cancer. What inner turmoil! With a pall of emotions all stirred up within, it was difficult to speculate or concentrate on one thing. But in the back of my head there was one thing that was certain, one thing that rang out; time was not my ally.

In my self-absorbed agony I forgot Anna was with me. She did not inquire about the visit and I was hesitant to confide in her. This was a private matter. I was dying. It was not news I wished to broadcast.

Looking at Anna I smiled warily. Finally, I decided to confide in her because she could be trusted to hold a confidence. Her hand gently touched mine. She understood.

All the way back to the office I sat silent, crouched against the front seat of Anna's car, entangled in shock and reality. The air was heavy with stillness. No words could have comforted me. "Here we are" broke into my anguish and signaled our arrival. My movements were slow, unwilling to face anyone. I was afraid that if confronted, I would lose control, the tears would gush, and somehow everyone would know that I was dying from cancer. Anna and I hugged tightly in lieu of words, then parted.

A strong front was required. Breaking down and making a spectacle of myself was out of the question. Calling up my self-control, I put on my cloak of concealment—an unapproachable attitude. With shoulders erect, head held high, and stern countenance, I hurriedly walked towards the plant, not looking to the left or right but straight ahead. This callous veneer which camouflaged my true feelings became the first layer of the protective cocoon I had started building.

Back at my office, I collapsed on the chair that swiveled under my weight. I stared through the same window that earlier brought me lightness of heart, but this time I was lost in sadness. The news that I had cancer continued to send shock waves through my body. I cradled my face in my hands as I sought to keep composed and control the hysteria that was lurking in my throat. My heart cried the Psalmist David's words: Oh Lord, you know what I long for; you hear all my groans. My heart is pounding, my strength is gone and my eyes have lost their brightness. Do not abandon me, Oh Lord; do not stay away, my God! Help me now, oh Lord, my Savior.

A spring of silent tears flowed uncontrollably down my cheeks. The journey I had originally embarked upon had taken a dangerous turn. I wondered if I had stayed home in Trinidad, my birthplace, and not ventured to the United States, would I have suffered this fate? There was a feeling of loneliness as my head rested in my palms. Mamma would have called that position "propping sorrows." If Mamma or Daddy, my grandfather, were alive I would rush to Trinidad so I could be comforted. They not only had ways of making everything around seem all right, their calming influence was infectious. I felt so very alone.

My thoughts traveled to the tenderness of my childhood. How I missed Daddy and Mamma and wished they were around to soothe my sorrows. My tears increased, not for my situation but for the deep loss I now felt for them.

"Oh, for wings like a dove, to fly away and rest. I would fly to the far-off deserts and stay there. I would flee to some refuge from all this storm." The Psalmist David once again captured my true feelings. If I could turn back the pages of life, there would not be the problem of careless inattention to my health. Oh how I wished it was springtime in Trinidad, early spring, early years, young and healthy years. Physical and mental escape is what I wanted because what I now faced was no heroic call to action, with rewards of glory or "atta girl" for work well done. To live, I had to develop a strategy for survival, rally my cause; but most of all I had to persevere.

Up against life's whirlwind, my peace had been yanked apart, wounding my spirit. Moreover, my faith in God the Creator was about to be put through its greatest test and I was filled with fear—fear that was sharpened by the realities of cancer. How could I be strong and resolute in this state? How was this situation going to work out for me? Where was God in all this? Where was the divine intervention? Why didn't He protect me from myself, from this horrible disgrace? Where was the God of my childhood?

In the frivolity of my youth, my sister Leah and I used to sit on the gallery chairs and scream at the top of our voices, each trying to out do the other. Breathless and exhausted, we would throw ourselves cat-spraddle onto the polished hardwood floor, but still full of laughter. My eyes swelled with water and I wished I had a private place where I could beat my chest and scream at the top of my voice and release the pressure that was building within my heart. Pride kept me restrained. There was a need to pray but I could not concentrate. Disappointed with God, I could not focus on His goodness or promises of deliverance.

Thinking about recent events, everything began to fall into place. The headaches, fatigue and listless feelings were now understandable. Cancer had circled my heart and was pumping life out of my veins. No wonder I felt so tired and run down all the time. My body was nutritionally deficient. There had to be indicators. This cancer did not happen overnight. No illness does. The body, like any machine, gives warning signals, but I had ignored its red lights. I felt negligent and became filled with vexation. Self-blame, a feeling of unfounded guilt, became an instant blanket, covering me with chastisement. Cancer, the spirit breaker, had started its destructive plan.

I had a habit of documenting any variances in my health. I was good about that. As far as I could tell, there were no drastic changes in my health. Minor changes, yes. For instance, my menstrual cycle: the flow was heavier and now lasted seven days instead of five. Cramps, bloating and headache accompanied this. This was expected. It was probably, after all, time for my biological change. So to me, there was no need to worry. Was anything else overlooked? I combed my memory for answers. In the past, I had only experienced occasional headaches, but recently my head had been hammering away at me to pay attention. Growing accustomed to incidents such as this, I acknowledged this dis-ease by taking aspirin. Ignoring the cause, just treating the effects. Yes, there had been signals!

I recalled my visit to Dr. Kanagaki on March 28, 1989, because of a slight, non-painful swelling of the right glandular node, the area between my thigh and abdomen. Dr. Kanagaki agreed that the gland was slightly enlarged and referred me to a specialist the same day. After a thorough examination, the specialist assured me that everything was fine and there was no need for concern because the gland was not in a grape-like formation. He detailed glandular changes, then advised me to follow up with him if there were any changes. I left the doctor's office relieved that I was OK. Gradually, the swelling went down and there was no need to make a follow-up visit.

In retrospect, I should have noticed the telltale signs. But who pays attention to lakes with small ripples? It's the raging rivers that catch our attention. Before April 17, 1989, often my feet and face were noticeably swollen when I awoke in the morning, but it tended to go down during the day. There was also a slight change in the consistency of my bowel movements that I did not think was drastic enough to be concerned about. Dis-ease kept knocking for me to pay attention.

Deeper introspection brought even more alarming signals to mind. During the winters of 1987 and 1988 I was undergoing tremendous negative stress at work. This was accompanied by bouts of flu. The usual home remedies—fluids and rest that had brought me relief in the past—had not worked. My illness had grown increasingly worse, forcing me to see my physician. On both occasions, I was told that I had bronchitis, and antibiotics were prescribed. In spite of being ill, I forced myself to continue my daily work activities, but I became so sick that I was compelled to take to bed. It is my habit to push myself, and my determination to practice this habit played havoc with my body. My immune system was so weak that even after I completed the prescribed medication, the cough, aches and tiredness continued.

On one occasion, the doctor increased the strength of the antibiotic I was taking because the previously prescribed medication was not doing the job. How distinctly I remember the siege of coughing spells that seemed to linger for weeks and the difficulty shaking the sick and tired feeling. Evidently my resistance was low, and my body was crying out, but once again I paid scant attention to my body's dis-ease and so I kept pushing and pushing myself. Oh, if I had only taken the time to rest my mind and body, exercise, eat properly and rebuild my body's strength and not push myself, maybe—just maybe—I would not have been in this position. As I thought about this sequence of events, I remembered the age-old saying, "Prevention is better than cure."

As I looked back, other incidents began to creep in to my mind. August, 1988, just eight months before finding out I had cancer, something occurred that is unforgettably tucked away in my mind. I was vacationing with my family in Germany. Our travels took us from Frankfurt through scenic and romantic places like Heidelberg, Fussen, Munich, Rothenburg and many other beautiful cities. Of all the cities, I remembered Rothenburg the best. Rothenburg is a small cultural paradise with narrow cobblestone streets passing by picturesque buildings that have jolly yellow and red facades. As we strolled through the square, crowds of people from all walks of life were gathered to watch a play that commemorates the siege of Rothenburg by the troops of Tilly during the Thirty Years War of 1631. Hand-carved puppets enacted the famous story of "Meisetrunk," master draught, a local legend of how the town's mayor saved Rothenburg from barbarians by drinking a huge tankard of beer.

Rothenburg is a gorgeous city. It is romantic, with so much history and so many different cultures, and I was there with my family enjoying it all. My daughter, Danielle, and I walked through the narrow, spotless streets holding hands and taking in the sights, while William played photographer. The weather was beautiful, the air clean and the warm breeze gently massaged our faces as we paraded up and down the hills and in and out of scenic attractions. As we took in the sights, we talked about how much we missed Robert, my son, and wished he were with us. He had chosen to stay home and enjoy the company of his friends, the "posse," instead of vacationing with "parents," as he put it. Captivated by the enchanting beauty, I was caught off guard as the dull menstrual pains that I had grown accustomed to lashed out without warning. In spite of the sick feeling, I was determined not allow pain to hamper this idyllic vacation.

During the afternoon, while visiting the specialty shops carrying fine crystals, steins, fine leather goods, and many other items, the pain grew increasingly worse. Gradually my body became overwhelmed with excruciating pain. It had taken center stage in my mind and body. Increasingly, I found I could not summon the strength to enjoy the scrumptious food or the frivolity that surrounded me. Not wanting to ruin my family's pleasure, my discomfort was kept private. I took two Pamprins, hoping for quick relief. A martyr I am not, but I was determined that I would not burden my family with my distress. So, underneath my ingenuous facade, pain and clenched teeth became my constant companions.

For years, I had heard women share stories of menstrual cramps accompanied by pain, headaches or vomiting so severe that they had to take to their beds. Although I empathized, I could not identify with them because throughout the years I had been free of menstrual cramps. But towards the end of that day, as I slowly maneuvered the streets in Rothenburg, the pain in my stomach became so severe that it halted my activities for a while.

By the setting of the sun, the pain grew to such unbearable proportions that it drained my total reservoir of tolerance. I distinctly recall the intense pain in my head that seemed to be synchronized with every movement of my body. My head felt as if it was weighed down by a ton of bricks that benumbed my sensibilities. So excruciating was the ache in my head that the slightest movement, even the vibration of a closing door intensified it. Nothing seemed to ease the discomfort except complete immobility and silence. Additionally, my legs were drained of strength as if I had just completed a marathon, rather than a casual day's walk. My tender bloated abdomen palpitated with pain as if I was in labor when clots were discharged.

I recall desperately looking in my purse like an addict, for a pack of additional Pamprin or anything to ease my brutal discomfort. The hotel bed covered with a fluffy, peach-colored, down feather duvet, was inviting and comfortable, but it did not provide any release. The night, instead of bringing rest, brought increased anguish. I vividly remember quietly slipping out of bed so as not to disturb William who lay in sweet slumber. Just another Pamprin, I thought, would certainly numb my pains. Trying to be quiet, I slowly eased my frame off the bed and toddled to the bathroom. My body was so racked with pain as I entered the bathroom that I froze. Forced to take comfort on the cold, plum-colored ceramic floor, I lay paralyzed, hopelessly clutching my stomach as I groaned. The coldness of the bathroom tiles acted like an anesthetic for my pains. After a while, relief came, allowing me to returned to the warmth of the bed.

The following morning my deliberate movements signified that something was wrong. This drew worried looks from William and Danielle. Concerned, they inquired as to what was the matter. No longer could I hide my discomfort from them. Furthermore, I was out of Pamprins and needed to find a pharmacy to buy something to subdue the dull pain that was still lingering. My face and feet were noticeably swollen but I attributed this to the previous day's walk and changes in my diet.

With time I had grown accustomed to bouts of physical changes and my gynecologist had given me a clean bill of health the previous month. That erased my concerns and gave credibility to my belief that I was getting older and going through the change of life. Yes, there had been signs aplenty! How I wished I had paid closer attention to my body's disease and heeded the call to change. Now, regrets set in like hot coals upon dry bush.

3

The Tilt of Balance in My Life

The real purpose for existence,
Is not to make a living.
But to make a life-a-worthy,
Well-rounded, useful life.
                                    Author Unknown

Cancer was found in my endometrial lining (the membrane lining the uterus)! I kept remembering the one thing I was desperately trying to forget. Try as I may, it would not let me alone. Cancer, a soul stealer and a spirit breaker, had taken me hostage with much ferocity. It placed me in the midst of a long psychological battle for survival and uncovered Pandora's box of negativity wide open. Feelings of doubt, despair, death, fear and other psychological distress took wings and attacked my waning hope with zest.

I tried giving myself words of encouragement in an effort to convince myself that everything was going to be OK. Except, instead of understanding and peace, a new wave of hopelessness ricocheted throughout my body leaving deep splinters of weakness and emotional instability. Cancer continued its chastisement. The carousel of negativity would not stop and let me get off! It began jerking me around, playing devious faith-weakening games, pitting fear against hope, pessimism against optimism, reality against untruth, death against living. I longed for peace and hope. Surprisingly, I found this to be elusive and deceptively complex. It was not a matter of mere thoughts, wants or words, but of faith, passion and deeds—behaviors that I was currently lacking. "Oh, Precious Lord, take my hand, lead me on, let me stand. I am tired, I am worn, I am weak. Hear my cry, hear my call, hold my hand lest I fall." Cancer once again brought tears to my eyes. Somehow, somehow, this soul hunter had to be defeated.

Unwilling to be submissive to this disease, I struggled to understand what was going on within my body. What had rendered my immune system ineffective? Most of my body's powerful defensive network for combating disease had left me helpless and vulnerable. What had gone wrong? Wisdom told me that this biochemical breakdown had not happened overnight—disease does not happen overnight. I was casually aware of some of the documented external and internal factors that cause cancer such as: carcinogens in the environment, chemicals, radiation, viruses, the sun, hormones, immune conditions, inherited mutations, smoking and diet. Were any of these factors direct contributors to my illness? Several close family members had died from this disease. Probably, I had the propensity towards cancer.

I took my clammy head in my hands as a nagging thought kept resurfacing; prolonged internalization of negative stress breaks down the immune system and leaves the body vulnerable to catastrophic illness. This was fact, not probability! Was this the case with me? Recently I acknowledged the need to reduce the negative stress in my life, but I did not follow through with change. Was it too late?

An anesthetic was needed for the pain that now gripped my heart and would not let go. It was cutting deeply at me two ways, physically and mentally. Philosophic reflections surfaced and I was drawn to remember that pain is part of living. It is life's volcano awakening the dormant soul, taking it to unparalleled heights that otherwise may seem impossible. It is an uncompromising challenger and the greatest of teachers. Pain is sometimes better than laughter, for it has a cleansing influence on us.

The pendulum marking time seemed to increase its swing as I mulled over things. In my heart there was a desire to live. It held me; it was overpowering. I can be victorious over this cancer. I want to live! These gallant words were not empty, neither was this desire to live due to a flash of lightning or some religious conversion. It was not because of my children or my husband, although I wanted to be there for them. Even when I first found out that I had cancer, my natural reaction was: "I am going to live, I am going to beat this." The majority of people, who are ill, want to live. They do not want to die. It is innate to all; this will to live is common to all organisms.

Oh how I needed hope, but hope seem to mock me for I knew without it I would die. Clearly now, I saw things with my mind's eyes and with a firm hold on reality I tried remembering times of bravery, when my faith was severely tested. None came to mind. If only I could recall some detail that could give me a vision of hope, how comforting that would be! I questioned: What is hope? What is will? What is faith?

Where do they come from? Do they come from one's inner self? Or do they emerge from one's spiritual, religious or philosophical beliefs? Do they come from observation and experience? And how can I hang on to them if surgery, chemotherapy or radiation fail? Who or what could I turn to in this my greatest need?

Soberly I remembered it was faith that connected me to God and brought me hope and freedom from worry. And faith, I was called to remember, is not exclusive to religious or spiritual people. Each person, the scriptures state, is given a small portion of faith. The child jumps with faith towards his father even though his arms are not outstretched, believing that he would be caught. In the past, I chose how much faith I wanted to exercise based on my mental and emotional stability or instability and the pictures in my head. Oh, if only I could succeed in holding onto my religious beliefs, and act on those beliefs, then I could have a stronghold on hope.

The teachings of my elders, inner strength, determination and faith in God, would be strongholds in the days to come. I had nothing else to hold on to. I was dying—I had to be brave. But true bravery consists not in merely wanting, thinking or wishing but in deeds. Isn't "faith without works" meaningless? I could not put all my faith and hope in physicians and medicine; these could fail and if these failed, so would my hope and my will to live. I had to believe from the depths of my heart that I could beat this cancer, for out of my heart, I remembered, springs forth life. Yet I felt lonely, tired and old. After much contemplation and with supreme effort, I found the will to pull energies together and resolved to help myself. This decision in itself brought me unspeakable relief.

Peculiarly calm now, and wondering how I should proceed, a sudden, desperate resourcefulness seized me, forcing me look to myself for answers. When we visit the physician we have to share our symptoms in order to be helped. Answers within myself were needed in order to help myself. In the past, I had been a keen competitor when it came to my personal and professional life. More so now than ever, I had to implement this same bullishness in my fight to live. I refused to leave my destiny to others!

A spectator in my own life, my existence had become so real, I could actually reach out and touch it. Putting an end to pensive observation, I concluded that if I could only succeed in renewing my mind and win the head game and stop feeding my fears, I could somehow actively participate in my healing. "If you want to find the answer, first look at yourself. Challenges that come your way are for you, not for the other person." Mamma's wisdom once again rang out loud. A bold plan was needed. Unwilling to leave matters up to chance and in a frantic effort to help myself, I made a determined attempt to proceed with the excruciating examination of myself and my environment.

I must emphasize that the decision to proceed with self-examination was a matter of feelings rather than a strategic plan, of survival instincts rather than reason. It was an urgent need to free myself from the demons that bound me, to release me to think and act anew. This traumatic experience was calling forth new adjustments of my mind. As I proceeded with earnestness of purpose, I agreed that I could not pick and chose areas that made me feel good and ignore the painful areas. This gave me an uncomfortable feeling. Nevertheless, I was willing to empty myself in order to be refilled with new visions of life.

First, I acknowledged that I was a divine being, created with a purpose, who was loved and in love. Surprisingly though, as I examined myself, I realized that I was going through the routine emotions of living, but not really engaging life. The pure essence of my existence, what I was all about, was missing. I did not know my purpose or my place in life. In fact, I was not looking for them. So much of what I had become was acquisition—picking up behavior patterns along the way. This was not an unnatural process, but my adult development was not a conscious effort on my part. The defining aspects of my behaviors and the path that I had become accustomed to were different from my intent. With an attitude of indifference to my life, I unwisely abolished ownership for my development. Inadvertently, I realized that over the years, other people began to play an important role in my own validation. Relatively unimportant things and issues got in the way of what I should have been, and blocked my involvement in what I could be. Slyly, my false values began their seduction and cunningly my inner joy was squelched, resulting in mental, emotional, physical and spiritual disharmony. This whole scenario compromised my evolution in being a whole person and left my spirit languishing.

The truth about myself had to be clear—my liberation could not be left ambiguous. This new revelation left me with an uneasy feeling. "Truth," Herbert Aptheker states, "advances through the detection of error; error is detected through reason and through science." (And, others may add, through revelation.) "To one who thinks, there is no greater service that the detection of error."

With humility I acknowledged my critical errors. Painful though the revelation was, it was indeed the beginning of understanding and the foundation upon which change is built.

Determined to be honest with myself, and acknowledge the truths that surfaced, the slow and cautious process of self-examination continued, and my place of employment, where I spent most of my time, produced a stream of answers. Mine was a dynamic environment! Daily challenges were met head-on, but most importantly, it was very stressful, oppressive and demanding. Although goals were attained, the process of achieving them was inefficient. Some days there was little time left for real productive work and for meeting critical deadlines. I agree that initially, aggressive activities must be implemented to improve productivity and efficiencies and I relished the discipline of wise, hard work. But eleven- and twelve-hour days, Saturdays and some Sundays, were the expectation and became the norm. Such excessive demands infringed on my personal life and prevented me from meeting family commitments. This resulted in harbored resentments and elasticized edginess.

To be sure, work environments are never idyllic and uniform structure is not always the goal. But at work, contradictions were the norm, values and morals were tested daily and, consciously or unconsciously, spirits were systematically battered and broken. That was the daily fare in my work environment.

There was definitely a gulf of misunderstanding between what I expected and what was. My strong sense of right and wrong, respect for others, and my thrust for social change and justice accompanied me into the work place. This saddle of well-being, became a yoke of resistance because, as it turned out, the business environment was not the place for personal altruistic idealism. Underneath its ingenious facade of performance and rewards, lay a volcano of replete capitalistic economics. This misunderstanding became a snare and a disillusion for me, and my environment became a vigorous competitor.

Since I had held different positions during the previous ten years I thought I had a fair understanding of corporate behaviors and business politics. I expected high ethics in the work place. I remembered how deep-seated work ethics, character, and reputation were lodged in my grandfather's business backbone. I had attentively listened to him as he bought and exported goods from Grenada and developed real estate. He was a kind man who had integrity. Ruthlessness, insensitivity and callous manipulation were never part of his business reputation, nor were they ever taught in college—at least not to women. Never in my wildest imagination had I conceived the hostile and manipulative environment that was lurking to grasp my will. And I refused to build the thick layer of skin that experience offered.

It started so innocently. My entrance into this environment was filled with naive virtuosity, initiative, a thirst for learning, a willingness to contribute, visions of accomplishment, and expectations of rewards and growth. With defiance, I refused to put on the armor of callousness, the protective gear necessary to successfully compete in this environment. I must confess that I never subjected my decision to the analysis of responsibilities or resulting ramifications that corporate America dishes out. Surprisingly, cursing, loud talking, manipulation, lying, cheating and autocratic domination were the way of doing business. These values produced internal turmoil because they were in direct conflict with my Judeo-Christian beliefs. The nibbling at my spirit had started.

The challenges I faced could be singularly defined. I was at fault. There were inconsistencies in what I was called to do and what I did. I entered this work marriage reluctant to conform to the norms, hoping to change the other partner. Instead, it got the better part of me. But in spite of all these challenges and on the surface of things, I would have to acknowledge that I had a very successful career. My achievements though were wounded by tragedy. Can you imagine the amount of energy and emotions I had to constantly exert in an environment of dwindling ethics? I was "successful," at least by society's standard, but at the expense of my health.

As the purging continued, I reflected over that period of my life and tried to understand what had gone on. Calmly and clearly, I realized that God was no longer the center of my life. In the past, trusting God gave me hope and enabled me to face life fearlessly and without worry. Now, the freedom, inner peace, joy, patience, wisdom and understanding that this relationship once produced was greatly diluted. I became a chronic worrier, no longer waiting upon the Lord, and I lacked time "To consider the lilies of the field as they grow." Entrapped in circumstance, forgiving and forgetting became harder. Subsequently I gave meaning to hurtful events, holding firmly to them although they weighed me down. Given the behavioral changes, I should have been alerted that I was on the wrong path—but I wasn't. I felt comfortable with the superficial contentment and somewhat enjoyed the tough, unforgiving veneer that masked the true me.

A crafty change had taken place. My forgiving nature, easy smile, quick laughter and inward joy that were always part of me were gone. I allowed the circle of ego and environmental circumstance to distort my cluster of values that was so much a part of me. The persistent discontent with my work environment continued and it became quite evident that I could not let go of the clandestine inward strife that grew from my daily experiences. Negative stress, thoughts and emotions; anger, resentment, anxiety, frustration, distrust and hate hung onto me like parasites and became entrenched in my behavior. In response, my stomach churned at every perceived distasteful remark or what I thought was an unjust act. You see, my uncontrolled thoughts became the standard for my behavior. Disease is not a punishment, but in most cases, a result of our behavior.

As much as I would like to blame mutated genes, people, environmental factors or my family's propensity towards cancer for my present malady, and contentious as the arguments might be, for or against, I could not absolve myself as a contributor to the disease I was now battling. Mentally, I wanted to distance myself from the deductions I had made and firmly lay blame somewhere else. Self-conscious of what people might think, I began to query the wisdom of my deductions and conclusions. I tried to vindicate and distance myself from blame, but supporting evidence to the contrary flooded into my head. I recalled times when I was nervous or scared. Often there were unconscious, uncontrollable physical manifestations to these emotions. I did not say to my body: O.K. body, I am scared, start the biochemical process of: diarrhea, constipation, sweaty palms, tenseness, headaches, weak knees, sleepiness, insomnia, heartburn, nervousness, overeating, lack of appetite, resistance, submission, fight or flight. Without conscious participation on my part, my body reacted to what was going on in my head.

I reasoned: Does heartburn stop although one continues to be upset and worried? No. The acids continue to do their destructive work. I remembered the difficult times I had falling asleep when my mind was not at peace. I had to mentally and physically make changes in order to get a good night's rest. What happens if one internalizes negative stress: worry, pain, resentment, grief or hatred for years? The mind does not say; "This is detrimental to your body. I will send some neutralizers to dilute the excessive chemicals that have begun to break down your immune system." Yes, an antacid will soothe the burning effects of heartburn. And yes, pills will put you to sleep and, yes, medicine will ease the pain in your head and calm your nerves. But they only treat the effects not the cause. Only when one acknowledges the need for change, and makes the required changes, then and only then will the body begin to regenerate.

Drug and alcohol addicts, prostitutes, workaholics and gluttons are not the only self-abusing sufferers in life. We tend to focus on the obvious sufferers and are shocked when someone commits suicide, gets seriously ill, walks away from a high-paying position, packs up and leaves one's family, or sees one's self imprisoned in one's own wallpaper. We do not understand the depth of one's internal suffering or the demons that secretly possess others, ravishing their minds and bodies—

sometimes death being their only way out. Often we refuse to believe that our loved ones are unhappy and need to engage life and follow their life's purpose instead of just living. I was beginning to understand the connectivity between the mind and body and could not argue with the scientists or the scripture; they are one.

Forced to concede to facts, additional convincing was not needed that my mind and body are one. You see I know myself; no one knows me better than me. The seeds from my habits had taken root. It was the natural consequence of neglect. My state of my mind determined my attitude towards my health. The suicidal emotions—hostility, anger, fear, resentment and hate that became barnacles on my behavior do not differentiate in their destructiveness. They are all poisonous to the body! Oh how deceitful the heart is! Love and hate, anger and peace, resentment and acceptance can all abide side by side, giving a false sense that everything is all right and there is no need for change

Unwilling to break the code of circumstance and have a relationship with myself, the changes in my behavior over the years caused me to deal with life strictly on an emotional level instead of harmoniously: spiritually, mentally, emotionally and physically. Often my responses were reactive, my words curt and cutting rather than contemplative and pleasant. This inhibiting physical alteration was not only in direct conflict with my disposition, but it was debilitating to my collective bodies. This tilt of balance caused disharmony within myself. With time, this discomfort was no longer an occasional experience. It had become ingrained in my everyday activities. It is a dangerous and treacherous illusion to believe work efficiency and good health can be sustained in negative stressful environments. The body is incapable of self-rejuvenation under constant abuse. I was cognizant of this but I disregarded the possibility of becoming ill.

Under the pressures of work and personal obligations, I blindly but expertly, began courting negative stress. The constant battles and long hours wore me down. There were too many long days and short restless nights. Countless mornings I awoke with a marked crease in my forehead and soreness from clenched jaws, left there by the night's subconscious stresses. I had placed myself in a position where I was receiving more from life than I could handle, therefore my body revolted from my extreme demands. I distinctly remember the tight and burning sensations that ran across my shoulders as I sat and listened to tirades in the work place. How clearly I remember the effortless irritability that knocked patience out of the way as I engaged in daily work activities. The emotional treadmill I was on, powered by ego, had increased to a dangerous pace.

Although I had reached my threshold of unhappiness in my callous work environment, I foolishly stayed on, accepted additional responsibilities and took extra potent doses of negative stress. The side effects were fatigue, worry, skepticism, frustration, disenchantment and feelings of victimization. The fight and drive that characterized my work ethic had begun to diminish. No longer was I jumping out of bed with enthusiasm to go to the plant. In a real sense, my career had become nothing but a tiresome job. And my daily activities were reduced to android-like motions of repetitiveness. Desensitization did not happen overnight. Too busy, it had slowly and insidiously crept upon me.

As I reflected upon my life, I recognized the contradictions. Arguably, many would say that I was a successful fast-tracker who was compensated well, so what's the issue? But in the aura of this success, I did not ask who I was. "There can be no happiness if things we believe in are different from the things we do," Freya Stark clearly states. I was definitely in the wrong place, trying to do the right things. Quitting the position had often crossed my mind, but I hung on, seduced by the approval of others.

This attitude of unhappiness prevailed and as I thought, that is what I became. I shook my head and smiled as I remembered that during that period, I routinely geared up to do daily battle. I must have lost my mind!

I was also aware that my thought is the fuel, the chemical activity that powers my behavior. An emotion, I knew, is the assignment of a thought. And every time I got upset, my physical body secretly produced additional and detrimental quantities of adrenaline, cortisol and endorphin that increased my heart rate and constrained my breathing. When this chemical process goes on within the body, lymphocytes needed for a strong immune system are severely impaired. These excess chemicals, instead of working for the good of my body, work against it. This process was initiated every time negative stress was internalized. Under these conditions, my killer cells that fight disease became inactive and the systematic breaking down of my immune system was underway.

With time, I adopted a conciliatory attitude toward things I disagreed with and which were not in accordance with my ethics. I assumed a firm position of indifference, shackled my potential and began courting disaster as I lost the lightness of life. In doing so, I discarded my initial teachings, thus throwing caution to the wind. In fact, I forgot not only what I had been taught but also, most of all, I did not listen to the tugs of my heart.

At work, I began to anticipate problems and react based on this anticipation, instead of making thoughtful assessments steeped in reality. Mountains were made out of molehills; I crossed bridges before they were built, worried about tomorrow, and did not live for the moment. "Oh, what peace I forfeited, oh, what needless pains I bore."

Unintentionally, over the years, I had become mentally, physically, emotionally and spiritually bankrupt. This combined with the potent mixture of fatigue, stress, grief, resistance, hatred, disenchantment, disappointment, resentment, lack of exercise and improper diet were toxic to my body.

Cavalierly I discounted my body's dis-ease: tiredness, irritability, shallow breathing, colds, tightness in the shoulder muscles, heart palpitations, tenseness and headaches. Instead of viewing these symptoms as warning signals, I believed they were part of doing business. They were nothing to worry about. Now my body was under siege. The smoldering, direct link of dis-ease had manifested itself into a full-blown disease, cancer—a consequence of my behavior.

Negative stress, this unwanted self-assertive villain, had slowly and systematically broken down my body's immune system and left it open and vulnerable to disease. The obvious mental and physical strain that this negative cohort exerted on my body was frightfully illusive. Faced with this catastrophic illness, I found myself worn out, broken down, burnt out, over-booked, tensed, and just plain tired. I was always thinking and doing, constantly running and giving without stopping to refuel; constantly performing on empty. Life's treadmill had turned into a tightrope on which I was performing a delicate balancing act. As I shook my head with sadness, I concluded that my current destination was not worth the trip.

My past had become an uncompromising teacher, the greatest teacher. "Dear Lord and Father of Mankind, forgive my foolish ways! Reclothe me in my rightful mind." Daddy's distant voice rang strong in my ear. God created this world in six days and rested on the seventh. In the New Testament, on many occasions, Jesus, the example, was found resting. Even with this knowledge, I kept pushing myself relentlessly without sufficient rest. I had become a reluctant student of life. If I had only realized that it was indispensable to my well-being, I would have made life-saving adjustments.

Sad to say, I was no longer myself. What I had become, was not what I had intended to be. I had created an environment that was slowly strangling me and had constructed a culture of complacency concerning my well-being. The result of self-examination was cruel, but kind at the same time, a real eye opener, an era of awakening and enlightenment. Soberly, I concluded that if prolonged internalization of negative stress helps breaks down the immune system, then the opposite must be true. Positive thoughts and behavior and healthy living could aid the immune system. I was persuaded and wanted to change. Antionio Gramsci appropriately wrote: "The most advanced thinker is he who understands that his adversary may express a truth which might be incorporated in his own ideas, even if in a minor way." My body and soul needed healing and restoration. It was essential that I learn from my adversary and past behaviors for the present and future molding of myself.

I was willing to change in order to live. I took ownership for my behavior. It was the first step in healing. I was willing to be transformed by the renewing of my mind. If it were not for the tyrannical call—the spawning of cancer—I would not have been moved to participate in this personal growth.

"Like any other major experience, illness actually changes us. How? Well, for one thing, we are temporarily relieved from meeting the pressure of the world head-on... We enter a realm of introspection and self-analysis. We soberly, perhaps for the first time, think about our past and future... Illness gives us that rarest thing in the world—a second chance, not only at health, but at life itself!"

Dr. Louis E. Bison

4

Understanding

And you shall know the truth, and
the truth shall make you free.
                    John 8:32

Unyieldingly and with infinite patience I worked to find understanding. This I believe is the wisdom of life. But let me assure you, self-examination is very exhaustive and terribly hard work. Sober thoughts and questions accompanied by clarity continued to flood my head in an awkward layman's way. I was drawn to ponder: Often illness is psychologically separated from our emotional, mental and physical behavior. We absolve ourselves as contributors and look externally to ourselves for a cure. Additionally, we are more versed on the workings of a computer or car than with the inner workings of our precious bodies. How then can we fend off disease?

I tried to relax myself. The galling yoke that kept me harnessed so many years was loosened but not thrown off. It would take time to reinvent myself and get my life back in order. Thankful that my heart and head had spoken to me and I had listened, I felt a peculiar calm. The burning pain in my heart had stopped as soon as I applied my energy to finding understanding. And through understanding, I gained much wisdom. Acceptance of reason and truth were no longer just relevant but imperative.

I began to look closely at how wonderfully I was made! This intricate, complex machine not only has the awesome ability to succinctly store and retrieve information, and the capacity to analyze and reason, and the capability to seek truth and accept it, it has the unique, innate ability to change. Now, instead of pain, excitement oozed from within my heart. The realization that my destructive behaviors exacerbated my propensity towards cancer and that my circumstance molded me, provided me with an overwhelming sense of relief. Without a doubt, I believed that: I am the caretaker of my body and I have the innate ability to change. Fortified with these truths, I concluded that being healed from cancer was possible. I was excited with the process of discovery and the opportunity for renewal.

In the past I had heard people enumerate their maladies with satisfaction. Some seeking pity, others boasting of their recoveries while still battling the same or different illness. I emphatically state: Disease does not in any way shape or form promote growth. It is a crucial wake-up call for us to pay attention and change. This fact should be obvious. Yet, in daily practice, we seem to overlook this simple and important point as we egotistically and insidiously push ourselves to the brink, tethering with dis-ease and disease. In addition, I had disregarded my propensity towards cancer and did not exercise preventative methods. I heard my difficult wake-up call, a call I hope, that was not too late. Forced to make extraordinary changes, the poignant question for me was: how could I develop and implement logical, life-saving solutions and not allow the frenzies of cancer to influence my behavior and decisions?

Oh how I longed for the days when I was healthy and laughter was easy. Memories taunted the present but the past could not be relived. I knew what had to be done. Proper living had been ingrained in me as a child. But distracted by the business of life, I strayed from my understanding of the scriptures and did not treat my body as a temple. It took this catastrophe for the scales of my eyes to be removed and viewed with new light, the preciousness of life—for without life, there is nothing. With this in view, I decided with great determination to make positive changes. I decided that my primary function was to reconstruct my behavior and environment that would be conducive to a long, healthy life.

While undergoing my mental reformation, which I decided would be implemented in behavioral and environmental changes, I felt tempted to hold on to time-consuming extracurricular activities, things that gave me a sense of importance; several board positions and overwhelming volunteer work. For me, there could be no holding on to impetuous wants, the change had to be drastic, immediate and permanent. I was pressed with the urgency to differentiate between necessity within reason, and egotistical desires.

Taken back by introspection and decision-making, I was unaware of the lateness of the day. The sunset emitted a red glow as the clouds grasped the last of its warmth. I could hear my husband's voice: "Red sky in the morning, sailors take warning. Red sky at night, sailors' delight." It was time to leave for college where I was working towards a second master's degree. As I packed my briefcase, I shook my head as the tears flowed once again. "Was it all worth it?" Eleven- and twelve-hour work days, Saturday meetings and even some Sundays; eating and praying on the run, recycled office air, lack of exercise, college three nights a week, missed doctor's appointments, personal and family responsibilities, conflicting values at work, harbored resentments, unhealthy eating habits, internalized grief, and not enough time for trivialities and laughter. Something had to suffer. Yes, my health! Mamma would have said, "If you don't rest, your body will find a way." I shook my head with regrets, thinking that it might be too late to rectify the mistakes I had made earlier.

5

A Sister's Heartbreak

It is in loving, not in being loved,
the heart is blessed:
It is in giving, not in seeking gifts,
we find our quest;
Whatever be your longing or your need,
that give;
So shall your soul be fed,
and you indeed shall live.
                    —Author Unknown

I was first to arrive at class that night. Usually, I would be in a hurry and running late, but on April 17, I counted the stairs taking them slowly one by one. Periodically, I rested and glanced at the wooden stairs. They were worn from the constant treading of feet from those seeking knowledge. Although I had often experienced tiredness during the previous weeks while walking up those stairs, I took such exhaustion for granted. In short, I attributed my tiredness to too much hard work during the day. For the first time it dawned on me that all this time I had cancer, and it was slowly draining my life away.

Such thoughts followed me to my classroom. Meeting one of my classmates, who was sitting close to the entrance, I asked: "If your wife had cancer, would you like to know?" I wanted to use him as a gauge to find out just how much I should tell my husband. Since I was reluctant to share the news with William, I thought that if this man did not want to be told, then most likely William would respond similarly. "Immediately!" was his reply.

He had thrown me a curve. I neither wanted such a response nor expected to hear it. I desperately wanted some confirmation that my not telling William was the right thing to do. Deep within my heart I knew that William would like to know immediately, but I did not want him to endure my pain. My classmate was not as imperceptive as I thought. No sooner had those words come out of my mouth that he realized something was amiss.

"Yvonne," he asked, "Do you have cancer?"

"Yes," I responded as I fought to hold back the tears.

"I am sorry to hear that," he replied, reaching out to touch my hand. As quickly as he put out his hands, he pulled them back. We were mere acquaintances and he did not know how I was going to respond to his physical show of empathy.

"What are you doing here?" Showing his concern, he asked.

"Don't we have an exam tonight?"

"Yes we do, but you do not need to be here. The professor would understand and I am sure he would allow you to make up the exam."

In retrospect, I do not know why I went to class that night. Presumably, I was experiencing a form of denial and had an unconscious need to continue my routine. Cancer had such an impregnable hold on me that as I waited for the professor to arrive, my mind was frantic with conflicts, questions and possible solutions. The most poignant question was, whom should I tell first? Unclear on how to proceed and caught between the tag team of cancer and fear, I felt the urge to scream out and run from the pressure cooker of it all. If only I could get out of my body, rise above all, and leave everything behind. That, however, was impossible. I could not run away from reality. I had to pull myself together and draw on my internal resources. Unable to concentrate on the night's exam, I decided to go home. The knowledge of having cancer reverberated throughout my immediate environment, influencing everything that came into contact with me. I had planned to pursue my Ph.D. Now, my dreams, hopes and plans seemed tauntingly out of reach. I was faced with unexpected complications and interruptions. Though my mind was in turmoil, I had to get it together and clear my thoughts to meet the immediate challenges.

The idea of telling anyone about my illness was mind-bending and grievously depressing. In the past, I was critical of those who kept their illness private and didn't share it with their loved ones. But now, as I walked in their shoes, there was understanding. It's a hell you want to keep private. Fearful that the news would devastate William and the children, I chose secrecy. It never occurred to me to confide in my friends. People who have cancer are initially unable to think in a coherent manner. Abandoned by good health, they tend to be embarrassed and ashamed by the scourge of cancer as if it was some type of retribution. Therefore, emotions rather than reason seemed to prevail. I did not want to be bothered or expend the energy explaining my illness to anyone so I decided to handle my illness alone.

As I sought to separate emotion from reason and contemplate my situation, I began to size up the events and mentally make plans. My mother, who was spending her vacation with Leah and me, was due to return to Trinidad. Because she was scheduled to leave imminently, in two weeks, I had to tell her soon because the Department of Immigration and Naturalization Service was slow in responding to extension requests. She would have to file for an extension of her stay as soon as possible. I would not have to ask her to stay, but how was I going to tell her about my illness?

In all my travail and confusion the most overpowering question still remained, whom should I confide in? After much thought, I chose Leah, my sister, to confide in, keeping my secret in the family. She would be able to handle the news. She would understand my situation. She would never break my confidence and would only tell the persons I authorized her to tell. The rationalization was easy.

Leah, my blessed sister, was a nurse. She was my best friend, my confidant, prayer partner, and adviser. We had always been there for each other. Even as children, our souls seemed to be inextricably linked. Although Leah and I were only one year and a half apart, we experienced a special love. If no one else in the world loved me, I know that my sister would still love me. Our relationship was unconditional! As children we often dressed alike and were sometimes mistaken for twins. Even as adults we sometimes showed up at functions dressed alike without planning it. We experienced each other's joys and sorrows. As a child, if I was invited to a birthday party and Leah was not, I would take my goodies home so she could share my experience. She did the same. If she was punished, which was rare, I cried. We played the piano together and even shared the measles.

It was time for memories. They were kept alive, easy to retrieve. My thoughts began to run wild like carefree children. A smile engulfed my face as recollections of my childhood flashed in front of me, distracting me from my present reality. I remembered Trinidad, the isle of my birth, and Morvant, the town where I spent my formative years. There, Mamma and Daddy, our loving grandparents, brought up Leah and me instead of our playboy father and young mother. As I reflected, I concluded that the walks my sister Leah and I took with Daddy were the most memorable.

The early morning Caribbean air would hit me smack in the face when I stepped outside to accompany my grandfather and Leah, on our Sunday morning walks. Although the scents of the air varied with the time of year, the air was always so fresh and exhilarating. I just stood and sniffed it. A euphoric feeling came over me as the freshness of the air meshed with the strong, sweet scents of Lady of the Night perfume, solanacea flower and wild lilacs. The clucks, mews, caws, coos and whistles from native birds formed a unique blend of wake-up music, the loud kiskadee being the most distinct of the flock.

Sometimes I felt the effects of the soft trade winds as they blew steadily through the trees ever so gently. Leah and I wished they would blow harder as they sometimes did, so the ripe fruits could fall to the ground and we could eat them. How soothing were the memories.

It was with the idea of teaching that we took walks with Daddy. "These walks are not only for fun but for enlightenment, remembrance and praise," Daddy declared as we walked along dirt tracks that zigzagged over hills and valleys. Oftentimes he would take a stick and beat the overgrown grass: zootie, stinging nettle and the thorny pisant plants that hampered our path. "Look at God's magnificent handiwork!" Daddy expressed as he raised his arms to the sky. Leah and I dreaded getting embarrassed by our grandfather's antics, so we prayed that no one else saw his performance. "Look at the trees, the flowers and the fruits," and stopping all of a sudden he would point out the small dewdrops on the large dasheen leaves. "See, children, God is everywhere. He even made the dewdrops!" This fascinated me, and I wondered how they got there when it had not rained the night before. The drops looked so even as if each was dropped by one of Mamma's eye droppers. Did God also have a dropper? I wondered. Pointing to the drops, he continued his teaching. "This cannot be seen when the sun is out," subtly reinforcing the need to rise before the sun.

Daddy was only about 5' 9" but to me he was a giant of a man. When he took off his hat it revealed a full head of dark hair. But Mamma's hair sparkled with gray. His brown, rugged features were kind and his smile lines deep. Not only did his ambidexterity fascinate Leah and me; his one brown eye and one blue eye were equally intriguing. When questioned about them, he chuckled and told us that he was blessed and wonderfully made. A quiet peace always surrounded him and he never raised his voice or said a harsh word. His relationship with God was special and I knew he could protect me from anything.

My grandfather had an oasis of experience and knowledge that he willingly shared with anyone who would listen. He inspired and instilled in me a sense of living, of being alive and being a part of God's grand scheme of nature. "Lee and Vonnie," as he sometimes called us, "life is made up of events. Make the most of each and do not put too much on your plate. Never distance yourself from the land, it is life-giving. Grow a garden, but most of all seek God for yourself." He taught me to sense nature, feel it, see it, but most of all to respect it. "All these things, children, like all things, come from God."

Mamma attributed my grandfather's faithfulness and love for God to his life-threatening experience. She always related the story with candid reflection. It is told that Daddy was knocking at death's door with an unknown illness. To make matters worse, the best physicians on the island of Trinidad were baffled and could not remedy his sickness. Mamma believed that her husband's last vestige of hope was wiped out. With health swiftly fading, a group of Seventh-Day-Adventist prayer warriors, along with family comforters, came to visit Daddy, who at that time was a non-believer. It is said that these witnesses told him about God's love. The believers told him that The Creator is a miracle worker and a healer of mankind.

Mamma said that they convinced him that everything is possible with God. He need only ask in explicit faith. Faith, they told Daddy, was the core to healing and his relationship with the Creator. "For without faith," they said, "it is impossible to please God, because anyone who comes to him must believe that He exists and He rewards those who earnestly seek Him." Hebrews 11:6.

"Brother Greene," using grandfather's surname, "you must hold fast to the profession of your faith without wavering, for He who promised is faithful." Hebrews 10: 23. They told him that if he had faith as a grain of mustard seed, he would be healed. With shortness of breath and explicit faith, Daddy made a crucial decision. It is said that he openly asked forgiveness for his sins, then asked God to come into his life and heal him. That night, he secured his tenet with the Creator and made a covenant to serve him always.

The prayer warriors stayed with him during the night, praying and singing songs such as A Mighty Fortress is our God and Trust and Obey. They reinforced his decision by sharing miracle after miracles with him. They upheld Daddy with "the prayers of a righteous man availeth much," and "where two or three are gathered in His name, He is in the midst to bless. God is the same yesterday, today and tomorrow."

It is told that the signs of anxiety, fear and hopelessness were eradicated. Daddy's hope was renewed. There was rejoicing the following day as my grandfather took a turn for the better and from that day he began to build his personal relationship with God. Mamma always closed her testimony with, "Child, weeping may remain for a night, but rejoicing comes in the morning. Oh Lord, you turned my mourning into dancing. O lord my God, I will give thanks to you forever." My solid framework for faith building and faith testing had begun construction.

From an early age, I was keenly aware of God's goodness towards me and that His love and mercy were all I needed to take me through life. "Yvonne, don't forget to count your blessings," Mamma often reminded me. Then she would proceed to tell me for the hundredth time the story of my childhood illness. "Several months after your birth, you were hospitalized, seriously ill. Your kidneys were malfunctioning and you were swollen all over. The doctor's report was not good and we were scared that you would die, my little Vonnie. We petitioned God for healing because you were too young to demonstrate faith. Daddy and I interceded for you." She always ended with, "And here you are today, alive and healthy. You must give God the praise." My faith walk took on an early start as I, too, started building a personal relationship with God the Father.

What a balance Mamma was in my life! A woman of few words, she nonetheless encouraged conversation and self-expression. There were very few no's in her vocabulary but no was no and yes was yes. She infused me with pride, and taught me to be disciplined and self-motivated. Muzzie, as Mamma was called by her loved ones, did not waste words with idle threats. She often reinforced her expressions with actions. This self-reliant woman was well read and very learned in "home physicianing," as she called it. Frequently, she shared her learning with us and with deep sincerity and love implored us to take care of ourselves. She noted: "It is of the utmost importance that you notice changes in your body. Your body is like a car. It gives you signals before it is in need of repair. God is the great physician but remember that He created doctors. So, please, children, do see a doctor if:

There are changes in a wart or mole
Swelling of the feet and pains in the lower back
Lump in the breast
Glandular swelling and pain; more so if there is no visible sign of injury
Changes in bowel movements, prolonged constipation or diarrhea
Dry constant cough or bloody sputum
Changes in menstrual flow
Constant headaches, especially those accompanied by dizziness."

These were her basic warning signals, and she implored us to know them as we knew the palms of our hands.

Mamma's melodious soprano voice always accompanied her daily activities. The hymns she sang were effectively soothing. As far back as I can remember, my grandparents were consistent in their behavior and there weren't contradictions in their lifestyles. They did not hold us to higher standards than they held for themselves. What they taught in the home was what they practiced. Their teachings are still indelible within my heart. Although I may have deviated from the Seventh-Day-Adventist religion, after I left home, I never forgot their teachings.

I would never have imagined that my early teachings and memories, Mamma and Daddy's unquestionable faith in God, their sense of discipline, songs of praise, unconditional love and their commitment to a strong family would prove to be bastions of strength as I faced cancer.

Buoyed up by memories, I dialed Leah's home number and listened to her soft "hello" at the other end of the line.

My sister was endowed with a calming spirit and was accustomed to situations like this. "Hello, sis."

Leah's voice was full of excitement when she heard my voice at the other end of the telephone.

"Hello, my dear."

Hesitantly, I broke the news to her just before she left for work at a local hospital. Calm, soft-spoken Leah was distraught.

"Oh no!" she cried in disbelief.

Sobs immediately followed and the uttering of, "Oh no, oh no, not you, Yvonne. Not my Yvonne." Her voice was wrenching. The threads in this fragile weave had begun falling apart. For a moment, I admit, her reaction caught me off guard. Yes, the news was shocking but not once did I think of my sister's reactions. Leah had always accepted negative news with decorum and reserved emotions. Usually she would shed her tears privately, never wanting to share her sorrow with the world. She always came back strengthened and in control. I was taken aback by her response to my news. For many years I had seen her in service of others as she comforted and reassured distressed families and provided care for the elderly. The results were phenomenal. I was looking to this self-assured person for support and guidance. Instead, I had to reassure and comfort her. "Cancer was found only in the endometrial lining, Leah, not all over, I am going to be fine. Please do not worry."

This explanation did not reduce her sobbing and muttering of "Oh no, oh nooo, not my sister," her voice choked with emotion. It is impossible to describe the sadness I felt as my heart ached for her. Leah and I had made an inseparable pair. It was easy to understand her feeling of utter distress. Part of her was seriously ill. My sister had taken part of my pain and stored it in her heart.

6

Determined to Go It Alone

Let us be patient!
These severe afflictions,
Not from the ground rise.
But oftentimes, celestial benediction,
assume this dark disguise.
                                            —Longfellow

Tired, sleepy and alone, I fell into bed around 7:00 p.m. which was earlier than usual for me. Night belongs to sleep but it proved to be elusive. I twisted and turned, trying to find that comfortable position which often brought repose but it was useless. This restless mood was set beginning with the phone call from Dr. Baez.

As I lay between hope and fear, I tried blocking out the day's turbulent litany of events but they kept flooding my mind with renewed clarity and energy. This must be a dream! In the morning I would awake, only to find out that this entire episode was a horrible nightmare. Did Dr. Baez say I had cancer, or did she say that she suspected that I had cancer? I recounted our meeting over and over again, reviewing every minute detail and praying that there was a flicker of misunderstanding on my part.

Unsuccessfully, I tried to relax by harnessing my scattered thoughts and emotions and by taking deep breaths of air. My body was so uptight that I found it impossible to unwind. Anxiety and fear, my predominant feelings, relegated relaxation and sleep to a back seat. Counting sheep from 1-1000 and 1000-1 was a fruitless exercise. I even visualized the sheep jumping fences. As I lay on my bed, hungering for emotional tranquillity, I looked at my husband and longed to reach over and put my arms around him. I knew that he would respond by reaching out and hold me in his arms, but I was scared that he would feel my trembling body and sense that something was wrong. I still felt this driving need to protect him from my pain and anguish, so I resisted the temptation and did not touch him.

In the darkness there's always some light. The full moon became my only comforter as its glare illuminated my side of the bed and kept me company as I waited and prayed for sweet rest. I must have fallen asleep, because I was startled into consciousness by the ringing of the telephone. Glancing at the clock I noticed it was 11:30 p.m. Reaching for the phone I thought that it might be an overseas call, because we often received overseas calls early in the morning or very late at night. Such, however, was not the case. It was Leah on the other end inquiring about my state of mind.

"How are you doing, my dear? Are you O.K.?" The gentleness in her voice was edged with pain. Oh Leah, Oh Leah!. I could tell that my sister was shaken and seemed near tears as she spoke. Not wanting to disturb William, and to keep my secret a little longer, I got up and retreated to the guest room and continued the conversation.

"I had a difficult time falling asleep. How are you feeling?"

"Comme Ci, Comme Ça." Leah responded back in our native lingo. "In fact," she continued, "I cannot function, Yvonne. I have been praying for you since we spoke this afternoon. God will take care of you, sweetheart. Yvonne, please stay home tomorrow so we can talk." She understood the difficulty of my struggle.

The ringing telephone and Leah's statements jarred me into stark realization. I was up, awake and frightfully aware that the conversation with my doctor was no dream. The morning's call was a dreadful irony, a numbing and brutal memory. My body shook as I cried tearlessly. A resurgence of emotional turmoil embodied me as the gravity of my condition hit home. Talking about my illness with anyone but a medical professional was the last thing I wanted to do, but I knew this meeting with Leah was inevitable. I would have preferred to sidestep the issue for now, but Leah's request that I stay home was a matter of formality. It would have been useless to try to discourage her. Whether I wanted it or not, she would come over.

In the darkness before dawn, I laid in bed mentally preparing for the meeting with my sister. Unlike an ordinary visit, I contemplated our encounter and wondered what was her agenda. As I lingered in bed, I heard the familiar engine of Leah's car. Her early arrival was unexpected. It was her habit to stop at the Italian produce stand and pick up fresh fruit and vegetables on her way home from work. The clock told me it was 7:30 a.m. Leah had not made any stops this morning.

Haggard from a sleepless night, I slowly sauntered downstairs to greet my sister. Using the key we had given her, Leah unlocked the door and entered the kitchen. Her nurse's clothes hung over her body as if they were hurriedly thrown on. Her cheeks were tearstained and her eyes were red. My heart dropped with sadness. It was impossible to ignore my sister's condition. Oh Leah, oh Leah. My dear sister looked exhausted as if she had been through the wringer.

We greeted each other with the usual hugs and kisses but her hug was firmer and her touch to my face was softer. The sad change in her troubled me. I had seen my sister cry only a few times during our lifetime. One of those times was the day of Mamma's funeral. By nature, Leah was calm, and I was the emotional one. My tears flowed at the drop of a hat. As I looked at her, I was having regrets for causing her pain. This was too much, I should not have told her. I really thought she would handle the news that I had cancer differently. Now she seemed to be in a realm of pain and emotional uncertainty. We reached out and embraced each other again, as we broke into tears.

Leah, however, regained her composure rather quickly. With renewed steadiness and pushing aside other pleasantries, she immediately delved into the issue at hand.

"Have you told William and the children that you have cancer?"

"No. I had given the situation some thought and I decided not to tell them."

Her mouth dropped open and she looked stunned. "You have decided what? You must be joking. Look here, girl," repeating a common Trinidadian phrase with emphasis,

"I am contemplating scheduling surgery while William is on one of his trips to Germany." I did not want my husband or the children to be around when I have surgery. My statements appalled Leah even as I was resolute about my decision. At that time I felt it was the right thing to do. But as I reflected on these events years later, I saw how expertly obscured my thinking was.

"You cannot have surgery without telling the family, Yvonne."

"Yes, I can."

"Chuts, man. What's wrong with you, girl? I have never seen you like this." Leah's Trinidadian accent became more pronounced. She rolled her eyes heavenward as if seeking divine intervention. "You need us and we need you."

"I'm trying to protect my family."

"What do you think the repercussions would be if you were to die during surgery? Your family would be devastated."

"You are making a mountain out of a mole hill."

"Cheups." Leah sucked her teeth and with a steady look she

continued the dialogue. "I have seen complications during surgery. No one can predict the outcome. You are not thinking rationally, Yvonne."

Leah and I had always been gifted with the ability to reason with each other after deliberating the facts. We experienced very few disagreements during the years and raising our voices at each other was out of the question. I cannot remember disliking my sister at any point in our lives and I valued her opinion. Leah did not contemplate my resistance to her suggestions. She was taken aback but stood firm in her persuasion.

"Someone has to assist you in making this decision, you are not thinking right." Her voice was straining to be normal.

In retrospect, my line of thought was irrational but I guess I was trying to gain some semblance of control in my life. "I am fine. I know what I am saying."

"It is important that you tell your husband, Yvonne. He needs to hear it from you, not from the doctor, or from me."

"There's no need to tell him, at least not now," I replied, standing firm by my decision. Fear and uncertainty had smartly clouded my ability to reason. I remained unconvinced by what my beloved sister was saying to me.

After a reflective silence, we continued our conversation. Taking the initiative, Leah proceeded. "I know you love William and the children, and I fully understand your need to protect them, but for a moment, Yvonne, think, think of the children."

I was thinking of them. Leah persisted, hammering away at me as if rehearsed. She got in my face and assumed an authoritative posture as she spoke. With her left hand akimbo, she gesticulated with her index finger. Her voice assumed a different connotation, a no-nonsense firmness that she had never used with me before.

"Listen here, Yvonne, this is no joking matter. You will tell them." Leah's divergent tone and disapproving face propelled me to listen to what she was saying. Earlier in our conversation, I was hearing Leah and responding automatically. But now I was listening to what she was saying. The pain in her voice was distinct. The urgency in her voice was poignant. My secret was now becoming my chastiser.

"Think of Robert and Danielle. We have brought them up with love, understanding and faith in God. We have fortified them for times like these and they are much stronger than you think. This is their test! Please do not deny them this opportunity for growth, love and support. They need to experience the whole spectrum of life. Illness, pain and suffering are part of life's lessons; they are part of the maturing process. It is necessary for them to experience different emotions. You cannot protect them from everything. Yvonne," uttering my name with such tenderness, Leah continued. "it is imperative that they continue to grow emotionally. Look at us. Mamma did not protect us from life's realities. We experienced birth, saw sickness and knew death at an early age. This is life. It's reality! Please do not deny them this opportunity for spiritual growth, the ability to exercise faith in God, the chance to demonstrate unconditional love, compassion and the opportunity to build patience. Our family's strength has been built on support, faith in God and trust. Please, Yvonne, do it for them."

This leap of growth, this test of strength would be profoundly painful for my children. It was not the type of test I wanted them to experience. Not wanting to hear more, I placed my fingers over my sister's mouth. Removing my hand but still holding it, Leah sat in the chair next to me at the kitchen table.

"What do you expect? How am I supposed to react, Yvonne? You are my sister and I love you so much. I have been unable to function since I received your call. Oh, how I wish it was me instead of you. You have so much to live for. I told God to take my life and spare yours. You have so much to live for." Her eyes brimmed with tears. What a fulfilling request she had made—at that time I did not know that Leah would die on October 25, 1992.

I had no intentions of remaining isolated with the knowledge of my illness but I just was not ready to share it with anyone right now. My reasoning continued to be distorted, as fear continued its subverted manipulation of my behavior. Unconsciously I was hiding from reality by not sharing the news with my loved ones. This emotion, fear, was driving me into seclusion, and I wanted to be left alone without having any more discussion. I wanted to sleep, think and develop a plan on how to proceed.

But even as I felt that way, I wondered whether I should have allowed Dr. Baez to inform the family as she had requested. No, I thought, I made the right decision in wanting to tell the family myself. I wanted to be the first in line and in control of what was going on. Information was not going to be transferred back and forth without my knowledge. "Does the patient know?" "Are you going to tell her/him?" On several occasions, I heard those questions asked by friends and family members. In fact, I remembered keeping much information from Mamma when she was ill because I did not want her to be burdened by the seriousness of her illness. But in spite of that, in my own case, I was not going to be kept in the dark.

I relapsed into silence but I was assailed with thoughts of my family. Their support was vital to my recovery; it had to be a joint effort.

But I was scared to tell them. What a paradox for me! I was ready to throw in the gauntlet and retire but Leah was not ready to leave. She kept pressing me to make the "right decision," as she termed it. If anyone could convince me, Leah could. She knew how much pressure I could withstand. After a while, in spite of my reluctance, I became convinced. Her appeal to my better self became more plausible and I conciliated. I had as important an obligation to my family as I had to myself. Forced to concede to reason, I agreed to tell William and the children in my own time, while Leah agreed to tell our mother. What a cumbersome agreement!

My sister smiled warily as we hugged and said our good-byes. It was definitely not a smile of victory. As I looked at Leah through the window, shuffling to her car with her shoulders slouched, burdened by the yoke of my illness, I could not help crying out: "Oh God, help us!"

7

Dashed Hopes

Doubt makes the mountain which faith can remove.
Toledo Blade, January, 1931

Time appeared to be fleeting by and I had to inquire as to the date. It seemed as if I had lost several days when in fact, only one day had passed since I had received the news. In spite of the fact that I was now on a course indicative of trials and testing, I felt strangely subdued. Apparently the roller coaster ride left me calm against the knowledge that there was a threat on my life.

What were my next steps? Where should I go from here? The next step was to call Dr. Julia Donovan's, surgeon/oncologist office in order to make an appointment to see her. Dr. Donovan was the person who with the help of God was going to remove the cancer. I wanted the cancer out, the sooner the better. Get out the disease and I can handle it from there. At that stage of my development, I believed that having diseased parts of my body removed would assist in the rejuvenation of my immune system and prolong my life. Therefore, my behavior was appropriate for the time. Hopeful with the possibilities, I made the call with anxiety and bated breath. I was given a May 8th appointment. The telephone query left me stunned! You cannot imagine the shocked and disappointed feeling.

"What! Did you say May 8th?"

"Yes, I said May 8th," the voice on the other end of the telephone was assumable soft, but the message was stinging.

"But that's 21 days away."

"Yes, it's about that."

The date echoed in my ears as the sound bounced off my eardrums. May 8th seemed like a lifetime away. I was mentally unprepared for this delay. The news was unbelievable! I could be dead and buried by then! I had to wait approximately a month from the D & C to see the doctor. My case was critical. It was a matter of life and death. The receptionist did not have a chart on me. She did not know my history and was unaware of the critical nature of my illness.

Dumbfounded and horrified I whispered, although no one was in the room, "I have cancer."

"Oh, I am so sorry to hear that. Please try and keep your appointment."

That was not what I wanted to hear. I expected her to give me an earlier date. A shadow was cast over my optimism producing a suffocating effect. For a moment I was speechless as I struggled to gain my composure. My heart raced with fright as my body became peppered with fear. I was tempted to get an attitude and make demands and in the same vane, I wanted to cry and beg but I kept my composure and stifled these natural emotions. This experienced person did not understand that my life would be shortened by a month, if I did not see the doctor sooner than the date she had given me. Pressured by fear, patience was not the virtue I was willing to exercise. So once again, I tried to obtain an earlier date.

"Do you have any open slots sooner than the 8th?" I ardently pleaded with a strange mixture of anxiety and excitement.

"No. The doctor's schedule is full with office visits and surgeries," the receptionist said convincingly.

Gaining my composure, I slowed my speech and requested that she give me a call if there were any cancellations.

"There are rarely cancellations, but I will make a note of your request."

This course was uphill, uphill all the way. I felt so hopeless and at the same time I was shocked into the reality that life was continuing around me and the world did not stop to pay immediate attention to my condition and begin nurturing and making me a priority. The pressures from my illness and disappointment escalated as I hit my pillow with both hands, while crying out, "Oh no! Oh no! Please help me God."

Where is the break in all this unpleasantness? I was at the mercy of everyone! Why couldn't the doctor see me next week? Surely they could squeeze me in. This was an emergency! This cancer had to be removed as soon as possible. My memory quickly recalled Romans 8:28. "And we know that all things work together for good to them who love God." But where was the good in this delay? For now, the cancer was localized to the endometrial lining, or so I thought. Given the behavior of this aggressive enemy and its inability to stand still, had begun to rob me of my resilience to bounce back from bad news.

The images and perceptions I held in my head about cancer were filled with disaster—there were no good endings. It is without a doubt that my perception was tainted with fear but the images that flashed in front of me were real. Try as I may, I could not relinquish them. Effortlessly I had clung to the perceptions that cancerous tumors can grow to the size of grapefruits within a period of a month and others metastasizing throughout the body within four to six weeks. Conscious bondage presented itself and I gladly accepted it. Unable to contemplate and come to some rational conclusion about what was going on, I concentrated absolutely on perceptions. This kindled fear—fear of the cancer penetrating the lining and spreading. Silently I begged: You know what's wrong with me then let's not waste any more time in waiting around. Please see me, and prolong my life by operating soon. If I had to wait 20 days to see the doctor, when was surgery going to be performed, another month? "I would be near death's door then," I said aloud with anger and frustration.

The peace I had previously experienced was nothing but a snare and delusion. I anticipated everything falling into place, subsequently giving way to a smooth process—early visit to the doctor, successful surgery followed by a period of recovery. But this was deception based on past experience. I had fooled myself into believing that the process would be quick and smooth. However, I was wrong.

When I made the call I was upbeat, but fear took liberty with my emotions forcing me to bed devastated and scared of the possible consequences. My life was hanging in the balance and I was oblivious to everything—the doctor's schedule, her other patients, the availability of the operating team and room or anything else. This was my life! I just wanted this cancer out, now, not a month from now. Help me, Oh Lord! Please help me!

I was in the process of changing my behaviors from one dominated by emotions. But this—this surgery delay threw a monkey wrench in my process. I felt emotionally destitute as my spirit was flagrantly being battered. To make matters worse, burning embers from the initial conversation with Dr. Baez were still lingering. What upheaval of my bodies!

From history, I knew that the cancer was not going to remain stagnant during this period of delay. This frightened me even more. It was a known fact, it would continue its invasive behaviors and uncontrolled cell growth. In no time at all, the diseased cells could proliferate my body, killing and displacing the good cells that were left. What would be my prognosis if the cancer metastasized to different parts of my body? How could I find out the extent of the cancer, if I could not see the doctor until May 8th? This potential spreading had to be stopped soon. My expectancies were now confused. All optimism for early surgery had been dashed against the cliff shattering my hope.

I tried praying, but this invasive disease and its ability to destroy my life overshadowed my thoughts. Relaxed in the first stages of healing—truth and acceptance, I was caught off guard by this incredible resurgence of emotional turmoil. In a real sense, I was taking things in stride allowing the healing process to evolve. Still dependent on others for my inner peace, I called Dr. Kanagaki and informed him of my test results. I needed his assurance that I would be all right. He was touched by the information and inquired if a surgeon had been recommended. I told him that Dr. Baez had recommended Dr. Julia Donovan. He apprised me of the surgeon's competence and suggested that I have a colonoscopy performed by Dr. Paul Farkas.

I met Dr. Farkas on my first visit to him, the fall of 1984. He performed a colonoscopy on me that proved to be negative. I immediately called Dr. Farkas's office and was scheduled to see him April 20, 1989. Yes, yes! Thank God! I was relieved with the date; at least I would have some type of medical attention in the meantime. Unknown to Dr. Farkas, he was playing a major role in bridging my visit with Dr. Donovan.

A day had passed since Leah's visit when I received a call from my mother, her voice soft and low as if not wanting to disturb me. It seemed relatively clear that she knew I had cancer.

"How are you, my dear?" Her voice was hesitant. It was not the vibrant jovial welcome she usually greeted me with, teasing and sometimes disguising her voice, allowing me to play the guessing game. Not this time. Today she was quiet, waiting for my response.

"I am doing fine, how are you?"

"Cote ce cote la." She had opened up the avenue for me to broach the subject of the cancer by responding that she was only feeling "so, so" but I was not going to fall into the trap. I moved quickly and discussed extending her visitor's visa and she inquired about the necessary paperwork. I volunteered to take her to the Department of Immigration and Naturalization in Boston, knowing that it was a whole day's event.

After a brief silence and my unwillingness to discuss my condition, my mother broke the silence.

"How are Dani and Rob doing?"

"Very well, thank you."

"And William?"

"He is doing well also."

Distant good-byes were exchanged. Good, there was no mention of cancer. What a relief! This was not the time to pull her into the thick of things. Her hands would be soon full. But most of all, I did not want to rehash the events of the past days.

With time on my hands, I looked inquisitively at death, speculating in its finality and earthly void. Illness gives you time to think, and think and think. Central to my concerns, though, was the possibility of not being there for William and the children. I trembled at the thought. The idea of making the choice to give up and die before the fight kept criss-crossing my mind although I wanted to live. Light and darkness cannot occupy the same space, the same with life and death. The slightest consideration of death had to be immediately squelched. I wanted to live—I was going to live.

Two days off work were welcomed. I returned to work under disguise of well being and vowing not to divulge my secret to anyone, not even my dear friend Jan. Being in the thick of things would provide distraction from reality. Surprisingly, work activities no longer played a pivotal role in my life as it did three days ago. This was not a contemplative decision, but an immediate adjustment to circumstance.

What smooth passiveness had overtaken me! The long hours were immediately reduced. The environment was no longer tense, hostile or threatening. My defense mechanism was now unnecessary, the aggressive behavior was subdued, the competitiveness was put in check, the need to be correct and prove myself were irrelevant. Putting others first took a quick second. Nothing mattered but my life and the will to live. I smiled at the transformation. Change, I thought, can be instantaneous in life and death situations.

I saw Dr. Farkas on April 20. His tall stature and unpretentious look invites trust and his full beard hides the full effect of his warm smile. He looks like the outdoor type who might enjoy hiking and water rafting. This was someone I felt safe and comfortable with. Although this was only my third visit with him, I fully trusted and respected Dr. Farkas's competence. As I waited in the examining room for the doctor, there was no outward show of anxiousness but inside butterflies were nesting.

Upon seeing me, his greetings were with familiar warmth as if we had recently encountered each other. What relief! This doctor was a healer in more ways than one. I exhaled loudly, blowing air through my opened lips, trying to slow the beats of my heart as I waited in the examining room for the doctor. I was confident that if there were any polyps, non-cancerous growths or tumors, this doctor would find them.

The examination proceeded with detailed questioning as he listened to my lungs and stomach. He gently pressed on my stomach with trained fingers moving in a systematic fashion while asking: "Does this hurt?" Upon the conclusion of the examination, Dr. Farkas told me that he was scheduling a colonoscopy for April 24th.

"Is that date convenient for you," he asked with warmth.

"Yes it is," I enthusiastically answered. This is what I wanted, rapid proceedings.

No sooner had I arrived home Leah called. She was curious about my visit with Dr. Farkas and interrogated me intensely, probably thinking that I might hide details from her. Upon learning of the April 24 date—the date of the colonoscopy, she insisted on accompanying me to the hospital. Under normal circumstances, I would have welcomed her presence but not on the 24th of April. I calmly thanked her and declined her offer. To tell you the truth, it was a wasted statement. I knew better. Leah acted as if I never uttered a word.

"Honey, I'll take the day off. Just call and let me know what time I should pick you up."

Really, to argue at all would be fruitless. She was going to be there whether I wanted her or not. I smiled and shook my head in agreement as I said, "O.K., I'll let you know."

Although I felt I was mentally prepared to tell my family about my illness, I decided to delay the meeting until the outcome of the April 24, procedure. However, on April 22, 1989, I experienced sporadic bouts of hypersensitivity from being bounced around by waves of irritability. The slightest discomfort brought on tears, aroused annoyance and quiet anger----the pressure of my secret continued to manipulate my behaviors. Inasmuch as my husband and I are emotionally tuned into each other, he sensed something was on my mind but did not want to interfere, feeling my need to have some space and also knowing that I would confide in him when I was ready.

As the afternoon wore on, William and I decided to drive me to Connecticut to pick up an evening dress for that night's engagement. The buying of the dress was delayed due to my illness and the pending surgery of which he knew nothing about. During our casual conversation, William inquired about the basis for my irritability:

"What's wrong honey, you have been upset all day. Is something bothering you?"

Near tears I blurted out, "I have cancer."

Instantly, the tears swelled in my eyes as I regretted my statement. For me, the interest of the moment was the method and place, not the communication. It was my honest desire to protect my husband. The last thing I wanted to do was hurt him, but in my frustration to hold on to secrecy, the news came out, spontaneous and unrehearsed. "For out of the abundance heart the mouth surely speaks."

Enormous silence followed my news. Oddly, William kept quiet as if in shock and suspended belief. His hand gently touched mine. I sat motionless, not wanting to move which might signal my willingness for discussion. At such a time, words would be useless. I did not want sympathy or pity. The weekend passed without incident or discussion of the subject. William was reserved with his conversation.

No one can make clear to another
who has never had a certain feeling,
In what the quality or worth of it consists.
One must have musical ears
To know the value of a symphony;
One must have been in love one's self
To understand a lover's state of mind.
                                    —unknown

8

Two Cancers!

*The deeper that sorrow
carves into your being,
the more joy you can contain.*
                    Kahlil Gibran

Leah arrived early and drove me to Baystate Medical Center, her place of employment, and the place where the endoscopy procedure and surgery were going to be performed.

The colonoscopy that Dr. Farkas, an expert endoscopist, was going to perform would allow him to examine the inside of my colon or large intestine. It is a highly reliable method for determining the presence and severity of diseases of the colon. It can reveal details not seen on x-rays. Optimistic about the results of the procedure, I was convinced that the colonoscopy was being done out of mere formality: for ruling out, not for finding out. But per chance a polyp was found, I knew that Dr. Farkas would easily remove it.

In the meantime, Leah had ingratiated herself with the staff and colleagues, asserting herself as my intermediary. I hoped that she would leave and return at the end of the procedure. After she had taken care of the pleasantries, Leah and I sat silently in the preoperative area waiting for the nurse to start the IV. Occasionally I glanced at my sister from the sides of my eyes. She was silent, seemingly lost in prayer. Fear had cooled off sufficiently allowing me some peace. This was a reflection of my optimistic attitude towards the procedure. Prayer came easy this time as I asked God to bless and guide Dr. Farkas during the procedure. Not long after, the nurse started the IV I was wheeled me into the operating room.

I looked in fascination at the high tech machines and instruments that were in the room. Surveying the room, I was drawn to the long black coiled instrument (a colonscope) that lay on the surgical station. Dr. Farkas would be using it to perform the colonoscopy. Seeing it reminded me of the 'snake' that is commonly used by Roto Rooter tradesmen. I smiled.

Dr. Farkas and the nurse went about their business in a professional manner: checking instruments and finalizing the procedural details. The mood in the room was cordial as the doctor kept me occupied with small talk.

He told me to lay on my left side, and then I felt the soothing effects as Dr. Farkas slowly injected the anesthesia into the IV that had already been previously started. "Where did you go on vacation, Yvonne?"

"My last trip was to Germany."

"Germany, tell me about it."

There's no memory of my response. The procedure was painless as I felt the flexible fiber-optic telescope move slowly up my colon. Dr. Farkas's voiced interrupted the quietude of the room: "Here is something."

Groggy, I asked: "Can I see?" There's no recollection of Dr. Farkas's response.

My optimism proved premature as it was shattered upon regaining consciousness. Dr. Farkas invited Leah and me to an office not far from where the procedure was performed. Our wait was brief but it was a very anxious time for us. Dr. Farkas spoke distinctly and deliberately, his voice enhanced by the quietness of the room. He informed us that a polyp and a cancerous tumor were found in my colon. Although Dr. Farkas's presentation was calm, not to cause me additional worry; the vestige of fear penetrated my soul. For a brief moment, no one said anything. I wanted to climb back on to the gurney and sleep this news away.

I choked back the scream that lurked in my throat. Suffering was running a streak against me. Why was life playing an unpardonable and macabre joke on me specifically targeting my heart? Where is the mercy, the hiatus from all this pain, this acute trauma? There was sporadic involvement in the conversation as I felt myself drifting off as if purposefully wanting to sleep the results away. Oh how I was thankful for the pleasant effects of anesthesia. Dr. Farkas' voice awoke me and pulled me into the conversation as he informed us that the tumor looked to be in the early stage and was operable. Two cancers! This was my worst nightmare. This was madness! That's what this was all about, sure madness. These were my thoughts as I drifted off again.

My eyes opened to an unusual stillness. I stole a quick glance at my sister. She sat frigid and unflinching with a slight grimace on her face that deepened the one dimple on the left side of her cheek. Tears swelled in her eyes and her chin dropped to her chest in sadness. Cancer that had killed so many was after her sister with a vengeance! There are limits to one's suffering. Can I bear this? I wondered if I was getting more from life than I could bear.

"Yvonne, I shall see you on April 25th for your follow-up visit. If you have any questions before, please give me a call."

"O.K., I'll be there."

I searched Dr. Farkas' eyes for some reassurance but they remained serene. After small pleasantries, Dr. Farkas shook our hands and left, giving us a moment to digest the news and possibly shed a tear. I gazed at his back as he swaggered out of the room one leg slightly slower than the other one. The room was calm but the sting remained in the air. I was up, and ready to go home and sleep. Leah hesitated, in a distracted sort of way. There was a long conclusive pause as she sat still for what seemed to be an eternity.

I turned desperately to Leah, "Let's go," my voice was slightly slurred, not from the anesthesia, but from the oppressive atmosphere and wrenching emotions of helplessness. The silence that followed seemed so long. Then breaking the silence in what seemed anger and prayer, Leah gave an excruciating exclamation that frightened me. "Two primaries! Oh my God!" Charged with emotion, she turned facing me, stretching out her hand she stroked my face with much tenderness. How was I supposed to respond? I had to help my sister.

"You heard him, Leah, the cancer is operable. Let's thank God that the colon cancer was found out before surgery, not after surgery." I responded in a comforting voice. Leah took my hand in hers, gazed into my eyes and forced a smile of agreement but her eyes stayed sad. As we left hand in hand, harnessed with this new information, I couldn't help thinking, that daunting days lay ahead as cancer continued to drive me back to the starting line.

9

Sharing My Secret with My Children

I never knew a night so black
light failed to follow on its track
I never knew a storm so gray,
It failed to have its clearing day.
I never knew such bleak despair
That there was not a rift somewhere.
I never knew an hour so dear,
Love could not fill it full of cheer.
                                    Unknown

Exhaustion and the lingering effects of anesthesia took over and soon I was fast asleep. Night and my children had arrived by the time I opened my eyes. Up and fully awake, Dr. Farkas' statement hit me like a bolt of lightning that sent me further downward into an emotional spiral. "My God, help me, please help me," my words were muffled by the pillow that I held firmly against my face, not wanting my children to hear my cries. From every angle, there seemed to be a massive conspiracy! I was worse off than expected! Time for sharing my secret was pressing and came more quickly than expected.

Faced with a barrage of new doubts, questions about my survivability began to feed my fears. Within a few hours my life expectancy had taken a nosedive. Was this the dark time before the dawn? Or was my faith being tested? I knew colon cancer was deadly, and early detection and treatment were necessities for survival. My detection was early, wasn't it? Doubts hinged to my thoughts as my mind probed my weakness, fear, and began to work on it. I remembered two of my relatives had died from colon cancer. Now I was scared, real scared.

There are over 33,000 new cases of endometrial cancer per year with an approximate 17% mortality rate. On the other hand, there are approximately 125,000 new cases of colon cancer per year with an approximate 49% mortality rate. Colon cancer was hostile and unyielding! What was my survival rate now that I had two cancers? Had it decreased because of both cancers? Mentally I began to calculate and speculate on some insensible survival percentage.

My God, what would have happened if both cancers had metastasized? Two cancers! My body was hammering away at itself. Hope tried escaping out the window but I held on to it. Relief, I needed relief from this terrible burden I was carrying. Oh, how I longed for additional sleep, and wished the anesthesia was still affecting me so I could lose myself in oblivion and forget everything.

Struggling to suppress an involuntary scream, I took my head in my hands and began to search my memory for something, anything that could give me hope. If there were no hope, I would die. I needed something to hold on to. A flood of memories swept across my mind and I remembered Jesus' miraculous healings. He had done it before, He'll do it again: "Oh Lord do it again; Make a way out of no way. Lord, I know you can. You've done it before, please do it again." Although my anguish reached fever pitch, I kept comforting myself by singing the song penned by Henry Davis & Shirley Berkley. "Help me Lord, Relieve this pain. I know you can. You've done it before. Please do it again." I needed comfort.

The children, oh my children, they were to be loved, protected and guided, not pushed into the face of adversity by themselves. I did not know how I was going to calm their fears and soothe their spirits. No matter how skillfully I had mentally prepared, it was not enough. Probably I should I tell them about one, and soften the blow. Nervousness stepped in as I participated in my own nightmare. Compose yourself Yvonne, compose yourself, I gave myself words of relaxation. As a child in Trinidad, I had seen the clouds hover, and experienced stormy winds and rains lambaste the earth with their fury, but there was always calm after the storm. I longed for that calm as I prayed for strength.

Contemplatively, I thought of the children I had given birth to. Robert Edward, my son, was a 17-year-old Boston College-bound track star. His cinnamon brown eyes were always twinkling with laughter and warmth. My son has never brought sadness to my heart or a tear to my eye. "Hey mom," he would say loudly as he entered the house making unnecessary noise as teenage boys do. The neighbors called our home Grand Central Station because it was kept alive with the presence of Robert and his friends from varsity soccer, basketball and track teams of which he was a member.

The posse, Tim, Will, Trey, Mark and Kevin, Robert's buddies, were welcomed additions. I met their girlfriends, laughed at their exploits and dished out advice whether they wanted it or not. Robert, who always included, loved and respected me; how could I at the crossroads of his maturing life share a pending catastrophe with him. It would impair his excitement about attending college, his thirst to achieve. I had to be careful. He was one of my reasons for living.

Danielle, my special gift, only eleven years, was conceived after a miscarriage. What can I tell her? Her dependency on me, her willingness to listen and seek out my guidance would make any heart glad. I can remember her saying; "I am a good child, I listen to you, mom." Oh Danielle! Her soft touch, sincere innocent eyes always reinforcing her beliefs that I would always be there for her. Our long talks, laughter, tears, shopping and special shared moments. Robert was extroverted but Danielle was reserved, gentle and sensitive. Although she was on the cheerleading squad and took dance lessons she loved being around her family and would choose to visit with us instead of her friends. She had a passion for reading and would spend hours in her room reading. Her book discussions were an integral part of our daily lives. I could not anticipate her response to the pending news. She also was at the crossroads of her development. How could I shatter her world, her hopes and her security? Danielle needed continued stability in her life. She also was my reason for being alive. Thoughts of not being here for my children burdened my heart with sadness and propelled me further into the need to be secretive.

It was important for me to get it over with and tell the children before I changed my mind but most of all, before William got home from the office. I did not want to cope with three of them at once. I could not hold back the floodgates of tears as Robert and Danielle walked into the room in response to my call. It was impossible to keep my voice from breaking as the tears flowed incessantly. They began to comfort me without knowing my circumstance. Danielle's eyes swelled with tears as she looked at me. The children had never seen me in this state before. Everything held its breath as I tearfully told them that I had two primary cancers, cancers of the colon and endometrial lining.

"It is not as serious as it sounds," I sobbed and struggled with my words. They looked at me in apparent disbelief. Robert looked awe struck, stunned, his eyes enlarged. His body felt tense as he reached out and held me. He did not speak. He did not cry. He showed rigid self-control and I knew he was trying to be strong for Danielle and me.

Danielle, with eyes wide and shaking, she cried out, "Oh no," then burst into uncontrollable tears, her voice amplified with cries and her head shook with disbelief. How earth shattering their reactions! Danielle's hold on me tightened as if I was resisting her. I held her gently with one hand while stroking her head with the other. I needed to get hold of my emotions. They were now vulnerable, I knew I had to be careful. They will follow my cue. My children needed the strength they had seen me demonstrate in the past.

To give them reassurance, I said, "I am not crying because I am in any physical pain. It is very difficult for me to share this knowledge with anyone, especially those closest to me. I was reluctant to share this information with you at first, but Auntie convinced me that I should."

"Does Dad know?" Robert asked with concern.

"Yes, he does, son."

"How long have you known?" Robert continued his questioning.

"About a week."

"You should have told us before, Mom. You should not have kept it to yourself," Robert said with such maturity.

"Robert and Danielle, the pain of sharing this news with you was too great. I could not tell you before now."

We talked about love, faith, being there for each other and trusting in God.

"You are going to be all right, Mom, I know it," Robert stated with belief.

"I am going to pray for you every day, I know that God will answer my prayers," Danielle whispered breathless as she looked me straight in the eye.

"God will take care of you, Mom," Robert reinforced in his self-assured manner. "You are made of good stuff and you have a strong faith in God. You are going to be with us for a long time. You'll beat this, Mom." Remember, "If you think you are beaten you are!"

They were much stronger than I thought. Leah was right! They had been shaped by the family's teachings. The internal pain and fear I had previously experienced was my fear, my pain—my pain for my children. My anxiety died quickly and the dilemma that confronted me now seemed inconsequential. My imagination of what might take place was amplified based on my perception. I had to stop anticipating challenges. Bad habits are difficult to break.

Proudly I held my son and daughter as they kissed me good night. With arms around each other, they somberly retreated to their rooms. As I lay in bed, the vestige of nostalgia teased me. I remembered Danielle sneakily waiting until Rob was in the basement to turn off the lights and lock the basement door. She chose to do this only during the nighttime, knowing that Robert did not like darkness. She would jump with glee, filled with kinetic energy and shaking her hands in the air as Robert banged on the door begging for someone to open. "Open this door now, Danielle," he would demand. Danielle would not respond to his pleas, but giggled with mischief instead. "Mom, could you please open the door," he would shift, asking me, knowing fully well that she would not respond to his pleas.

Danielle would take off running as I opened the door aware that Rob would be in hot pursuit. Upon catching her, he would gently throw her on the floor and plant a kiss on her face that she wiped off in disgust, but with a smile. Rob would pin her to the floor until she promised not do it again. "Please let me up, Rob, I won't do it again, I promise," would be her girlish plea but she always continued to do it. She could not resist the pleasure in scaring him.

Robert was playful and enjoyed wrestling with his father. Often he would enter our bedroom, kiss me goodnight, then kiss his father. Catching his father off guard, he attempted to pull him off the bed. William always grabbed me, as he was about to fall on to the floor as if I would prevent him from hitting the rug. They would begin to wrestle, William using his legs to entangle Robert while still firmly holding on to me. I, in turn, would call to Danielle for help she would come running while shouting: "Leave my mother alone, let go of my mother, Daddy." She would feverishly work on her father's grasp trying to free me. What fun, what laughter! I laughed aloud as I remembered throwing a cup of cold water on William as he bathed and he doing the same. What memories! I wanted to make more—I had a lot to live for. It was time to rethink my whole relationship with life.

The sound of William's car engine broke into my memoirs. It was 7:30 p.m., when the front door was opened, then slammed shut. William's footsteps were hurried as he rushed upstairs, taking two steps at a time in his haste. My heart increased its beat, as I sensed something was not right. As if a light went off, I suddenly felt as if the impact of my earlier statement ("I have cancer") to my husband had hit home. Oh no, not now! Ruffled, I had no time to prepare. I was sitting up in bed when William walked into our bedroom. His face displayed grave concern. This confirmed my fears. I did not want to arouse sympathy but tears swelled in my eyes. Why couldn't it have waited a little longer? Once again, a well of uncontrollable tears ran down my cheeks.

The normal welcomes were unutterable as William moved towards the bed. My blessed husband dropped to his knees, held my hands and said: "I have asked God to afflict me with cancer instead of you. Not

that it was God's doing, but I am willing to be afflicted instead of you."
I quickly dropped to my knees and said: "Dear God, please strike out
that prayer; with your help, I know I can withstand anything." He
chuckled with surprise and looked at me with much compassion. My
husband who lamented over a paper cut was willing to sacrifice his
health in my stead. The moment was precious as we embraced and
cried. We understood. There wasn't a day that I did not feel William's
warmth and love. I thanked God for this special relationship.

Not wanting him to continue speaking, I said, "I have colon cancer
also." William turned his head and wept. I did too. Never did I see my
husband so broken up. Cancer was conspiring against this blessed relationship. "My poor wife," was his only response as he held me closely
and listened attentively as I shared the results of the colonoscopy. "I'll
be at your side, Sweetheart. I know you are going to beat this because
your faith in God is strong." After a while, I felt my tension melting. In
the coming months I'll need his caring support.

In honoring my obligation to Leah, and telling William and the children about my illness, I could now breathe easily. Filled with an inward
freedom, I was free to think and plan. The waters upon which I was
going to sail were uncharted. I, therefore, had to cautiously chart the
passage I should take. My family was counting on me and I was not
going to disappoint them. For once, my thoughts broadened and I was
able to objectively look at my circumstance. I wanted to live.

Later that week, I followed-up with Dr. Farkas at his office; there
he delved into the results of the colonoscopy he had performed on me.
He took time answering my questions, thus dispelling many uncertain-
ties. The keystone at this point, was truth. I wanted to know everything. He assured me that based on what he saw, the colon cancer was
operable. His eyes were trained and he was one of the best in his specialty. I believed him.

"What's next?" I inquired. "Can both surgeries be performed at the
same time?"

"I do not see why not, but I am not the surgeon."

He recommended Dr. Kasper, a general surgeon, and suggested
that I make an appointment to see him. Foregoing the long night's wait
I called Dr. Kasper's office that very afternoon. I was scheduled to see
him on May 11, 1989. The May 8 visit to Dr. Donovan was looking
good now.

10

A Convert to My Cause

Take your brick walls,
Lay them flat and make them stepping stones.
Yvonne L. Williams

The decision to stay home was easy. And so, I stayed in bed instead of getting up. I needed to restore some order to my life. What an experience! What rough riding! The last eight days were packed with unprecedented emotional tribulation and psychological warfare.

As I mulled the past events over in my mind, I realized that it was a good thing I couldn't get an immediate appointment with Dr. Donovan. To me, this was no coincidence; all things do work together for good to those who love God. But in spite of comforting reinforcements a day had not passed that I did not experience resurgence of emotional turmoil. It was difficult staying mentally calm and not be concerned about what was happening to my body. Although I prayed, read scriptures, gave myself encouraging words and had philosophical discussions with myself, I still had to fight and suppress negative thoughts. Having faith and staying calm in the face of adversity is not easy; it is a very difficult process. This psychological battle was taking so much out of me that often it seemed it would be easier to give up and die, than fight the cancer battle. But I did not want to give up. I desperately wanted to live.

Although this desperation to live came from the gut of my soul, I realized that I was noncommittal to my cause. This was a significant observation that came in a fleeting and powerful moment of reality. My mind was still in bondage—a slave to bad news, and the taunting connectivity between cancer and death. All the self-cajoling in an effort to separate the two was failing. I found myself caught in a web of illusion—believing that I had permanently severed the cancer and death connection. The condition of my mind had everything to do with the health of my physical and emotional system.

Reason now guided my will. The solution was not difficult, positive psychological sustainability was the challenge. I had a mind only I could control. I had an attitude towards a disease only I could fix. Contemplatively, I took a closer look at my family's medical history and concluded that there was a propensity towards cancer. Wanting to be a victor, I had to do whatever I could to change my environment and not be a victim to this disease. Often I had heard people talk about their family's propensity towards hypertension and diabetes but refused to make life saving environmental changes, thus making their propensities realities. Unknowingly, I had done the same. Determined to get back on the right track, a radical change was needed. In order to accomplish this, it was crucial for me to establish ownership over my plight, take control of my destiny and participate fully in my healing. I had to use my contemplative power and create new images within my mind—cancer is not death.

But this change—this healing process, this renewing of the mind, this purging with hyssop was not a matter of mere surgery, chemotherapy and recuperation. It wasn't just about survival or being alive with dependency on people, medication or hospitalization. I required a process for full recovery without the fear of a reoccurrence hovering over my head, scared that every ache is cancer. Supportive environments, loving family, competent physicians, new drugs, new techniques and experimental treatments are all necessities for battling catastrophic illness, but they are insufficient. I was now faced with a set of unique responsibilities.

Distracted by what was going on in my head, I overlooked the recent pain and tenderness I felt in the area of my ovaries. The pain was different from menstrual cramps and, instinctively, I knew something else was going wrong with my body. Questions and thoughts scampered in my head. Could the cancer have spread? Are there more than two cancers in my body? I had to know the survivability rate of people who had three or more cancers. My trembling finger dialed hospitals and agencies from Maryland, to Georgia, New York, Philadelphia, Massachusetts, and Connecticut looking for some type of survival statistics of people who had experienced three or more primary cancers. Absurdly, I was still relying on the experience of others to manipulate my outlook. "We do not keep statistics on people who have had three or more primary cancers. The mortality rate for those with three or more cancers is very high; therefore, there isn't any statistical value in keeping records. The few who survive, do not live past five years." The hopeless, staggering statements rang loud and clear in my head. I expected a firm grip on hope but instead, I plunged into despair.

Survivability began to weigh heavy on my mind. Yes, I had the unquestionable ability to forge ahead and yes, there were approximately 8 million people alive who had experienced various types of cancers. That was somewhat comforting but next to none of those 8 million had survived three or more primary cancers. People are different and handle situations differently; each experience is unique and each ability to compete different, I reasoned. But, stalked by the hopeless responses and the contending perceptions and images in my head, triggered new details of disaster. If there were three cancers, the odds for beating this treacherous disease were definitely against me. I should have let sleeping dogs lie and not made those calls. A little knowledge is really a dangerous thing. Faced with a new psychological stalemate, I continued to digest the enormity of the possibility. My face dripped with sweat as the possibilities of having three cancers began to covertly use me as its whipping pole.

Unlike all the other brash challenges I had recently faced, the fact that the survival was rare stopped me dead in my tracks. The sharp barrier that I now faced was more complex and presented many risks for me. I volleyed back and forth against the odds. Where would I get the mental and physical strength? Would I be able to rebound from this new psychological depression that was forcing its way upon me? What was going to make my case different from all the others who had walked in similar shoes?

Despite the evidence of what cancer could do to the body, my desire to live could not waver. But as much as I had an ingrained desire to survive, I also was confronted with a built-in worry factor. The one thing that daunted me through this period was my inability to completely block or discard cancer and its associations. This was my quagmire of fear, resulting in worry. Engaged in a contentious protracted battle, without any sharp bargains to make or shortcuts to take, I was determined not to acquiesce to the pressures of the struggle although I was now plagued by a resurgence of doubt.

With my faith shaken, I needed a stronghold of support, a shelter in the time of this storm.

My body had experienced all the emotional changes associated with the receipt of bad news. Now alone and abandoned to my own resolve, I needed the balm of Gilead, the peace that passeth all understanding.

When people are dying they will go to the ends of the earth to find a cure and do whatever it takes to find peace of mind.

People seek people and things that give them relief. I must once again share with you. The burden and difficulties of having two cancers were too much for me to carry alone. It is not about external support, but internal relief and strength. I wanted to be able to lay my secret psychological and emotional struggles and fear somewhere and in their stead, firmly grab hold of faith and hope. I had to draw on the source of my strength. The only thing I knew and believed that could give me hope and strength is complete faith in God the Creator and His son Jesus the Christ. With a philosophical shrug of my shoulders and throwing my hands up questioningly, I wonder if faith would really work in my situation. Yes, I knew all the scriptures, but my mind still inquired as to the reality of exercising faith. Blowing off the dust that so inconspicuously covered my religious beliefs, confidently, I decided to practice what I believed, and often talked about—trusting God explicitly for everything. There was nothing left for me to do but simply trust God. Taking a definitive stance, I decided to completely exercise the small portion of faith I was given. This was the crucial defining aspect for me, the turning point in my struggle.

11

Exercising My Faith in God

Prayer is not overcoming God's reluctance,
It is laying hold of His willingness.
Unknown

As I prepared my mind for faith strengthening prayer, I remembered that faith and perseverance go hand in hand. Prayer does not mean a world without pain. Sometimes healing takes time and it also comes with change. Faith is an action work. The scriptures state; "Faith without works is dead," and it is also "The substance of things hoped for, the evidence of things not seen." My faith in God could not waver because; "For without faith," I remembered, "it is impossible to please God."

Getting out of bed, I stood in front of the mirror and ran my fingers along my face and hands, closely looking at the lines on my face and the yellowness of my eyes. My hair uneven, broken from lack of nutrients. My stomach slightly distended. I looked old and fragile. Gently, I rubbed my arms as if I was rubbing new life into them; Daddy's miracle was on my mind. With faith I made the commitment to "Cast all my care upon God for He careth for me." Willingly, I accepted the challenge to steadfastly persevere. There was no turning back.

I believed without question that nothing was impossible when faith is exercised. I began talking to God the Creator as I touched my cancerous body. Numbers 23:19 states: God, "You are not man, that you should lie, or a son of man, that you should repent. You have said it, and it was done, You have spoken and it was fulfilled." I ask you God to touch my body and heal me with your healing balm. I continued to lay my case before my God. Your son has said in Luke 11:9-13. "And I tell you, ask and it will be given you; seek, and you will find; knock, and it will be opened to you. For everyone who asks, receives, and he who seeks finds, and to him who knocks, will be opened." "I will be strong and of good courage, I will not be frightened, neither be dismayed." 2 Samuel 22: 2-7. "For I know you will be with me through it all." Joshua 1:9. Yes Lord, I know You will be with me. I continued in prayer for a while.

At the conclusion of my talk with my heavenly Father, I thanked Him for healing me. Afterwards I fell into a deep peaceful sleep. Upon awaking I remembered that it was revealed to me through a dream, that I had ovarian cancer and that cancer had penetrated deep into the pelvic area, but my healing had begun. Surgery would be successful and the doctors would marvel at my recovery. I believed without a question, that my healing had started and the peace I had longed for now encompassed me and permeated my very being. Some may skeptically say that it was wishful thinking on my part, but I believed.

In the coming months, I understood that my faith would be tested. Therefore, I had to keep my eyes focused on the Father and His promises. Supportive behaviors had to be demonstrated. The mind cannot be fooled. I could not just speak or just contemplate faith. I had to believe and act upon it. "For as he thinketh in his heart, so is he." (Proverbs 23:7).

Surprisingly, this period of readiness had taken time, and could not be rushed. It was necessary for me to experience some of the body's natural reaction to calamity: doubt, fear, depression and sadness. Only when this phase had ended I was able exercise my portion of faith— the power of the will to change.

My psyche had to be self-correcting, charting my psychological course. I was converted to my cause without compromise. Infused with hope, my mental cobwebs that were so artfully wound around my thoughts and emotions began to fall apart. I realized that in order to implement the mental commitment I had just made, it was necessary for me to sweep away the vestige of all mental entanglement—I had to govern my thoughts.

First: I had to solidify the unprecedented challenge of acceptance— acceptance for my renewal and healing.

Second: It was necessary for me to confront my fears. Remembering that; "God hath not given us the spirit of fear, but of power, and of love and of a sound mind." And "Though I walk through the valley of the shadow of death I will fear no evil for God will be with me. His rod and staff will comfort me." In spite of all the reassurances, fear had become my constant companion, cunningly taking a strong hold within my subconscious and surfacing at the precise time. Like love, it is a natural emotion so I did not pay much attention to it at first, but I found it was trying to hold me emotionally imprisoned. Fear is like driving a car with the brakes on all the time. Eventually, the full functionality of the car will be impacted.

The same with our bodies! Fear hinders healing of body and mind and inhibits cures. My greatest challenge will be putting fear in check. It was necessary for me to reinforce my faith in God and master this natural emotion with genteel dominance.

Third: Understanding my options was of primary importance. My views of cancer were jaded by what I had seen and heard. It was essential for me to understand my options so I could forthrightly move ahead. My friend Debra Caporosa reinforces; "From nothing comes nothing," and "There's no victory without engagement." To win, I would have to be mentally prepared and armed with the right gear. Fighting is grueling business.

Fourth: The least I could do for myself was to exercise the art of self-love. This was not just a safeguard but the core to one's relationship with one's self and the Creator. Surprisingly, some type of morbid curiosity drew me to read the obituary columns, looking first at the cause of death or the memorial contributions. This sometimes gave me a clue to the cause of death. As was my practice, I opened the newspapers and read the obituary of a 39-year-old woman who died from cancer. Her accomplishments and achievements were numerous. Her involvement on different boards was remarkable! But the thing that struck me was the quote made by her husband: "My wife was a blessed woman, a saint on earth. She put the needs of everyone else above herself." That was key! This was not God's intent! Mark 12:31 clearly states: "Thou shalt love thy neighbor as thyself;" not more than thy self, not self-sacrificing, but as thy self. If only I had practiced the art of self-love and treated my body as a temple!

It is not only the use of drugs, alcohol or moral misconduct that destroy the body and mind. But simple things as loving others more than we love ourselves, overwork, lack of rest, improper diet, or internalization of negative stress. During many Team Building sessions at work, I was asked on several occasions to list the priorities and values in my life, with the first being the most important. In retrospect, the list was always the same: God, family, work, vacation, friends, money and the list went on. Never once did I list or consider myself a priority. It was always others or something. In retrospect, I was confused between self-love versus self-centeredness and in this confusion, I made some unwise sacrifices.

If I had made Yvonne a priority and not pushed myself unnecessarily I would not have been in this predicament. If I had only learned to say "No"—no to internalized grief and harbored resentments. I should have said no, and not have accepted additional responsibilities at work. If I had exercised self-love I would have said "no," I couldn't make that late unscheduled meeting. I also would have said "no," I cannot do it, I am too tired, and rested without the weight of guilt heavy on my mind and I would have put my inner drive in check and know when and how to put it into full gear.

Fifth: I had to decide that I wanted to live. Although I had a thirst for living and I believed without a doubt that I was going to survive, I had to make the decision that I wanted to live, for me, not for anyone else. I had thought about the commitment and even said the words, but they were uttered along with cluttered thoughts tinged with fear. The decision had to be clear and direct. It was my sole decision; a choice between life and death and it could not be taken for granted. The fight was singular, the decision absolutely mine.

The doctors would do their part by removing the diseased tissues and organs; combined therapies were possible, recuperative resources available, family and friends would always be a supportive cheering section but the fight was fundamentally mine. No one could will me to live or fight. My survival could not become dependent on the encouragement from others. The determination and driving force had to emanate from within. Faith and the will to live had to be part of my being, prominent in my every thought, especially in the face of isolation and silence. My determination could not be diluted, when I am alone at night with no visitors, no lights, no cheers and no encouragement, with only pain and doubts as companions. My decision to live could not wait for the doctors' prognosis, the appropriate time, or mental preparedness. Neither could it be based on the odds, or survival percentages. I could not incorporate them into my decision-making processes; if I did, the odds would be against me and the race would have already been lost. This matter of life's resolution could not vacillate between good or ill feelings or test results, for these will emotionally jerk you around and keep you on a perpetual roller coaster. I had to make the decision and stand firm no matter what. I had to be the empowered decision-maker.

Sixth: Cleansing mind of pent-up resentments was a practical necessity. As I stated before, honest self-scrutiny was difficult and self-interrogation disconcertingly revealing. But the decision to look within, and unearth grief, anger, dislike and resentment took moral courage and fortitude. I not only wanted to live, but to be truly happy—unencumbered by self-inflicted wounds. It was imperative for me to completely purge my mind of everything that was not restorative. Cleansing the mind was another main ingredient required for complete recovery. The healing had to be complete, both mind and body.

Fully cognizant that harboring any type of resentment was detrimental not only to the body but also to one's relationship with God, I could not continue internalizing divergent thoughts and expect any type of healing or cure. In the past, I discriminately chose which pain I wanted to carry and which persons I should shun. Hurt has a subliminal power over one and unconsciously I had carved out a place in my heart for resentment. This was my choice. Although I thought I had forgiven who had wronged me, I had not forgotten all. Seeing some of the individuals who had caused me pain or remembering the event ignited new flames of resentment. For to forgive is truly to forget, whatever the hurts were. If I did not forget, old wounds would never heal but continue to fester, thus affecting the ability to fully live and love.

Destructive behaviors are life threatening, because they slowly eat at the heart of our being— making way for illness. A clean wound heals quicker than one that is contaminated. The same could be said of a clean and uncluttered heart. The Bible states that if one part of the body is ill, then the whole body is ill. The ability to totally forgive and forget is one of the most powerful healing antidotes. A complete purge of the mind was necessary and it had to be immediate! This deadly illness had transforming power. It was teaching me things that my pride had not allowed me to learn over the years.

Seventh: I had to decide that I wanted to fight and believe in my fight. Although I knew that the odds for survival were against me, and at times it seemed as if everyone around me was dying from cancer, I had to continue my fight. When fear tries to grip my heart and hope seems to be fleeing, I had to continue the fight. My desire to live had to be unwavering even if I think that I am progressing but the test results say differently; when setbacks come while I am thinking all is well, I had to believe in my fight and continue.

Still, I had to believe in my fight and keep pressing on when staying in bed is easier than getting up. The fight must continue when the memory seems like it is failing, and even when the experts say they cannot do any more and dying seems easier than living. In spite of these, the fight must continue with faith, hope and mental prowess.

I knew that my energy could not be diluted, it had to be stove piped and channeled in the right direction. I also knew that I had to negate all possible distractions always thinking that even this shall pass, and keeping my eyes focused on my end goal, victory over cancer. I believed that no matter what the obstacles or setbacks are I would come through them victorious for this is part of the healing process. It is true that: Sometimes situations have to be slowed down to move ahead fast. Other times, it is better to break down in order to build up anew. At times, conditions get worse before getting better. Other times it is better to cease and rest for a while. No matter what the situation, I had to fortify my resolve, and be zealous about my fight and proceed in faith, for victory is always around the corner a few steps away.

Eight: It was critical for me to change my environment—breaking the chains of inherited and cultivated behaviors that were feeding these cancers. Unless I renovated my environment, it would be impossible to get rid of acquired propensities towards catastrophic illness. I had to free myself from my excessive, compulsive behavior—always pushing, doing, thinking. My response to daily challenges must change from subjective to objective. Recently, I had cultivated an attitude of disregard for proper diet. That had to change. Proper diet and exercise were ingrained in me as a child. In addition, I took pride in being able to perform on only five or six hours of sleep. This unreasonable demand on my body had to give way to self-restoration. I had to clearly define the elements in building a healthy environment.

Ninth: I had to practice the art of relaxation. Marcel Proust clearly states that: "Illness is the doctor to whom we pay most heed; to kindness, to knowledge, we make most promises only; to pain we obey." Forced to pay attention, I was now proactively setting aside time for relaxation and not allowing my illness to be the driving force. I thought that relaxation was a natural occurrence, but I was shocked into the realization that over the years I had slowly forgotten how to relax and the invigorating energy that it provides. This art of relaxation had to be reclaimed! Like any art form, it had to be learned, then continually practiced so that it becomes habit forming.

Tenth: I had to exercise my complete faith and trust in God. For me, this is the sole source of my strength and emotional stability. "Faith is the assurance of things hoped for, the evidence of things not seen." Hebrews 11:1. It is the belief in impossibilities. This was not a matter of transcendent faith-it had to be demonstrative faith! It is applying mental prowess and psyching one's self out to accomplish the impossible. Faith is setting the table when there is no food. Faith is trusting God where you can't trace Him. My relationship with God was based on faith and love, love for someone who had given me the life I was now fighting to keep. I had often failed Him, but in spite of my human failures, I know He cares.

I was determined to be a victor, not just a survivor! I wanted to chant. I wanted to beat the drums and send victorious messages. I wanted to sing loud victorious praises to my God. My battle had just started and I had to garner the strength to continue. There was no need for self-pity, round about talk or victorious guarantees. Demonstrative faith was needed for this victory. This unprecedented challenge was a practical lesson of faith and hope. It was left up to me, solely me, to chart my mental course.

During the next few days I went about the business of serious environmental change. My new cleansing diet was life saving. My daily exercise was refreshing. My voice was once again tinged with laughter. My relationship with the Creator was renewed and there was a positive spin on my thoughts and behavior. For the first time in several months my menstrual cycle came without pain. That, which once restrained me, now promoted me. I must share with you though. At first, it was very difficult to consistently swallow my medicine for healing but how transforming positive behaviors are! I felt the change. Others saw the change. I was becoming a new person. Old things were slipping away. Going about the business of renewal I remembered a poem I recited as a child.

If you think you are beaten, you are:

> If you think you dare not, you don't;
> If you think you'd like to win,
> but you think you can't,
> It is almost certain you won't.
> If you think you'll lose, you've lost,
> For out of this world you'll find
> Success begins with a person's will–
> It's all in the state of mind.

If you think you are outclassed, you are:

> You've got to think high to rise,
> You've got to be sure of yourself before
> You can ever win a prize.
> Life's battles doesn't always go
> To the faster or stronger man:
> But sooner or later, the man who wins
> Is the man who thinks he can.

12

My Visit with Dr. Donovan

Your attitude will determine your altitude.
Unknown

My steps hastened as I arrived early at Dr. Donovan's office for my
May 8th appointment. Slowly, I approached the office door, briefly
stopping, I viewed the sign on the door—suite #306, Dr. Julia
Donovan, M.D., Wesson Women's Group.

After filling out the pertinent forms and a brief wait, my name was
called and I was ushered into the examining room where I changed
and waited for the doctor's entrance. My heart skipped a beat when I
heard a knock. Dr. Donovan entered. Her smile was warm and hand-
shake firm as she greeted me and introduced herself.

"Good morning, Mrs. Williams, I am Dr. Donovan. How are you
feeling today?"

I wanted to respond with, "I am nervous," but I smiled and replied
with the run-of-the-mill answer, "I am fine, thank you."

Her personality was soothing, her smile inviting which brought me
relaxation. Unhurried, Dr. Donovan posed a few questions as she
looked over my chart with some familiarity. Her touch to my skin was
warm and gentle as she began her examination. The questions she
posed were direct as she patiently and methodically proceeded with
the examination.

I scanned her with intensity, taking everything in without being
judgmental, just accepting what I saw: Her small frame, fair skin,
reddish brown hair, the freckles on her arm. Her brown rimmed glasses were perched upon her nose and her lips perked to the sides when
she smiled and spoke. I looked attentively at the way she held
her hands, the white lab coat she wore and the way her name was
scribbled on it; her shoes; her wedding rings; the gold sapphire

bracelet that hung loosely around her wrist; everything. Fairly young to have such a remarkable reputation I wondered, hoping that she was as competent as was rumored. She continued to examine me; her skilled touch gentle.

Her questions were noninvasive, I felt relaxed and it became a smooth give and take. She inquired about my children. I did the same. Hers were very young compared to mine. Patiently, she continued her examination while questioning me and mentally taking notes. She relied on me to reconstruct bits and pieces of my life and past and present illness. There was instant pain in response to her touch.

"Does this area hurt?"

She returned to the area where my ovaries were located, gently and methodically pressing with trained fingers adding gentle pressure while asking, "Does this hurt?"

"Yes. I think I have ovarian cancer."

"Why do you think so?" Dr. Donovan asked her head tilted to one side as she waited for my response.

We had just met, I did not know her religious beliefs and I surely did not want her to think I was some kind of nut or religious fanatic.

"I was given a vision," was my response.

She nodded her head with understanding, not doubting my statement.

"I think I will have you undergo an Ultra Sound. The receptionist will schedule it for you."

The encounter and examination went well. The bonding was successful! What relief! I was ready for surgery and anxiously waited for the date it would take place. Dr. Donovan took off her gloves and began washing her hands, still no mention of the date.

"When is surgery scheduled?" My voice was full with apprehension, unable to wait any longer. Smiling, she indicated that we would discuss it in her office after I was dressed. The wait in her office was brief. I cannot remember the doctor's opening statements, but I know that she informed me that she would have to perform a hysterectomy, and would be assisted by Drs. Fischer and Lieberman. I was not paying much attention to what she was saying. The date, just tell me the date, I was thinking. I was not really interested in anything else.

Dr. Donovan continued by stating that if the cancer had penetrated the pelvic area, or if the Ultra Sound showed that I had additional cancer, then a radical hysterectomy would have to be performed. She proceeded by providing additional details moreover informing me about the pretests that had to be performed. I was O.K. with everything. Yes, yes, yes, just give me the date.

"I have scheduled surgery for May 17, here at Baystate Medical
Center. Admittance would take place on the afternoon of the 16th."

Taken aback I was ready to get emotionally worked up by having
to wait nine more days but I remembered the past events. My God was
in charge. I had to trust Him where I could not trace Him.

The visit to Dr. Kasper, the surgeon was five days prior to admittance. Dr. Kasper presented a very warm and inviting personality as he
entered the examining room after knocking. Although he was highly
recommended by Drs. Donovan, Kanagaki and Farkas I wanted additional details about his years in practice to which he responded with
satisfactory details.

Dr. Kasper questioned me about my medical history while reviewing my chart and turning and revisiting the attached correspondence as
if memorizing and cross-referencing the details. His methodological
probing questions assisted me in remembering the occasional dizziness
I experienced. Dr. Kasper assured me that both surgeries could be performed at the same time. "In fact, Yvonne, that's the game plan. Dr.
Donovan and her assistants will perform the hysterectomy, then I'll
proceed and do my part assisted by Dr. Hubli."

Dr. Kasper explained the procedure and informed me that a right
hemicolectomy would be performed in the area of the cecum (the
intestinal pouch which open into the ileum, colon and the appendix
veriforms). He simplified the details using the layman's lingo whilst
interjecting the necessary medical terminology and using a full sized
chart that graphically detailed the whole intestinal area to assist him.

I proceeded to satisfy my interest in several questions. How much
of the colon was going to be removed? Was the surgery complex?
Based on the test results, did he think that the cancer had penetrated
the Subserosa or Serosa (the first and second membrane of the of the
colon wall)? Satisfied with his qualified and honest answers, I was
ready for surgery.

13

Surgery—Three Cancers!

The feet must be washed in the blood of the heart;
before one can find the right path.

Hatha Yoga

Hospital Admittance

At approximately 12:00 noon, May 16, 1998, I headed out to the hospital where William and Leah waited. The pre-registration had taken place the previous day and all I had to do was sign some forms and pick up my admittance papers. Leah and William were silent as they escorted me to Room 217. Upon our admittance to the hospital room, Leah moved in a professional manner as she put my things neatly away, while William sat quietly, deep in thought. My husband and sister stayed a while, but they were asked to leave so that the preparation for surgery could begin. Their reluctance to leave was quite obvious as we said several good-byes. Finally, the nurse graciously asked them to leave.

May 17, 1989, William Recounts

I was going through some trying times, my loved one was stricken with cancer and I was scared. I did not indicate my fear openly because it was imperative that I show a strong front for Yvonne and the children; but I was going through my own private hell from the day I realized that Yvonne had cancer. I welled up with sadness at the thought of her being ill. I love her dearly and I needed her. I could not imagine life without her.

I do not remember much about May 17, 1989, the day surgery was performed on Yvonne, just the events pertaining to her operation. I do not recall what day it was or the time of year; spring I think, but I am not sure. I was oblivious to everything else. I was really focused on the events. Usually my mind wanders through all sorts of things on a given day, but on this day, I could only think of the operation while constantly praying for success.

As I recall, it began in the morning, really the evening before. It commenced when Leah and I checked Yvonne into Baystate Medical Center, one of the principle hospitals in the area. I felt somewhat comforted by the thought that it was a teaching hospital and therefore it was equipped with the latest technology. I think most people would have been in a quandary or in a very somber mood, but not Yvonne. She was light hearted and in good spirits with her usual witty manner. I knew this was not a put on. She was very relaxed because she believed that the surgery was going to be successful. Leah and I accompanied her to her assigned room after she had completed the usual forms required for admittance into the hospital.

We walked with her to her private room and she quickly transitioned into the role of hospital patient. They began almost immediately giving her all sorts of preparation medicines and I was quickly snapped into the reality of the situation. The packing of Yvonne's personal necessities for the hospital stay, the accompaniment of her to the hospital and the completion of the pertinent forms were all performed automatically—trance like. Now reality had set in. My wife would be going under the knife the next day. I felt as if it was a matter of life or death. We held hands and I desperately petitioned God in prayer. After some time Leah and I were asked to leave so the pre-surgical preparation could continue. Inwardly I did not want to leave. I longed to be there and usher her into sleep. Being alone can change positive situations into negative ones and I was concerned. I often wondered what that first night was like for her. Was she afraid? Did she sleep well? What were her thoughts?

My night was restless and my sleep was disturbed by the thought of Yvonne being alone and the fact that I had to be in the hospital by 7:00 a.m. I did not want to be late. Leah and I arrived at the hospital bright and early in order to meet with Dr. Julia Donovan. It was my first encounter with the person who was going to be the chief surgeon during the operation. I did not know much about her, only that Yvonne had a very strong trust in her and that she had a reputation as being one of the best. After introducing herself, Dr. Donovan took Leah and me aside and explained to us what was about to happen. Yvonne would be taken upstairs to an area where she would be prepared for the surgery. We could accompany her if we chose. Once she was moved into the operating room, surgery would begin. They were going to go in and examine her to confirm the presence of cancerous cells. If they found cancer, they would operate. Dr. Donovan would perform the first part of the surgery in the morning and it would take about four hours. The entire operation would take about six hours and Dr. Donovan would meet with us in between the two operations to let us know how things were going. This would be around noon. After that, Dr. Kasper would perform surgery in the afternoon. I was to let the nurses' station know my whereabouts at all times so they could find me if I was needed.

After the doctor left, events moved fast. Yvonne was soon placed on a gurney and wheeled up to the preparation room. Leah and I were told we could accompany her and we did. I held Yvonne's hand. I remember thinking how cold her hands were. I remember them being cold even prior to this day, but today they were especially cold. It felt as if life was slowly being ebbed away from my loved one. I held her hands tightly hoping to transfer some of my warmth. Although my heart was heavy, I really focused on my love for this wonderful woman, my wife. It seemed there was an unseen energy that channeled from her into me. She had strength from her belief in God and she passed that strength on to me. It was all coming through her from God. Leah must have felt it too, although we didn't discuss it.

Upstairs in the room where they prepared her for surgery it was all business. There was no connectivity, no personal relationships. The staff was competent and very professional. They accomplished their tasks while they accommodated us. I guess they were accustomed to this. Yvonne was still her usual outgoing self but I think she must have to be nervous, who wouldn't be under those circumstances. It would have been difficult for me not to be nervous. Pretty soon she was dressed in the part of one who is about to undergo surgery and a doctor came by and introduced himself. He told her that he was the anesthesiologist who would be administering the drug that would make her unconscious for the duration of the operation. I recalled my own minor surgery some years prior when I was given anesthesia and told to count backwards from 100. I think I got as far as 99.

At about 8:00 a.m., they wheeled her into the operating room. Although she was drowsy with anesthesia, we maintained eye contact until the doors were closed behind her. Leah and I returned to Yvonne's room for we were in for a long wait. We prayed right away and asked God to protect her and bring her back safely. My mother-in-law decided to stay at our home to be there for our two children, so Leah called to let her know how Yvonne was doing.

Both Leah and Yvonne had a strong belief in the power of prayer. I had my doubts, but my wife didn't. Yvonne especially had a strength I had never experienced in this kind of situation. She even calmly told me that I should go to work or go home and wait since there was nothing I could do at the hospital. "Please do not worry," she said, "nothing has ever been changed by worrying." For me, cancer had been a terminal illness. I've known several people who had it and I knew none who had survived it. None of them readily accepted their fate. They tried to fight it in certain ways. They gave up smoking as if this would somehow reverse their affliction. Others turned to miracle cures or holistic medicines. Some of them just gave up and accepted their condition and what they believed would ultimately end in death. Some displayed anger at their condition; anger at God or anger at the worldly conditions that they blamed for their affliction. I thought about these things as I waited at the hospital. Yvonne never displayed anger, or asked God why. I do not know if I would have held up that well being in her place. Leah worked at the hospital and she left to begin her shift. It was a long lonely day for me; I was scared, I was anxious and I cried inwardly as I waited in Yvonne's room. Sometimes I would go into the waiting room at the end of the corridor. Occasionally I would go to the cafeteria to get a cup of coffee or a drink, only to return to the room and wait. Time seemed to stand still!

Yvonne's private room gave me an opportunity to be alone to meditate and reexamine our lives. My faith in the power of prayer was not as strong as Yvonne's but I called on God many times during my hours of distress, and through it all my faith was strengthened. Over the years I had delved in many religious sects including Buddhism, Bahai, Baptist, Pentecostal and many more. I had been a humanist, an agnostic and an atheist. I was learning and searching for a philosophy and the meaning for existence. I had come full circle and was now a professed Christian. My wife and I have had many discussions about God, faith and other related topics, but Yvonne never forced her religious beliefs upon me. She always smiled and said something like, "I know He lives, He has never failed me yet;" or, "I will always trust him where I can't trace Him," or "Prayer changes things." Today, I needed that trust. I suppose some would read into this that God was strengthening my faith through the experience and I suppose He was. I would have preferred a different way to build my faith. Today, I had no doubt that God was at work throughout the entire experience.

The first few hours of waiting were agonizing. I could not concentrate on anything, not even the surgery. Shortly before noon, Leah returned and asked if Dr. Donovan had come by as she had promised she would. I told her that I had not seen the doctor since morning when she had first met with us. Noon was drawing nigh and I was anxious. Leah told me not to worry and after another prayer together, she left. Time passed and it was now 12:30 p.m. I thought: "In circum-stances like these, no news is not good news." But my anxiousness turned into fear. Time was no longer standing still and I did not see or hear from Dr. Donovan. I kept looking down the halls with anticipa-tion and my heart palpitated as I heard footsteps along the corridors, some of them now becoming familiar as the nurses walked back and forth.

I wanted to know what was going on. Why hadn't the doctor called? How was the surgery proceeding? I desperately needed to find out. It was now 2:00 p.m. but still no news. I inquired of the nurses about the status but they had no updates. I called and informed my mother-in-law who tried to calm my nerves, but how could I calm them in a situation like this? It was now 4:00 p.m. and I felt that something was wrong, dreadfully wrong and I would not leave for fear that the doctor would stop by and not find me. Leah came back several times and inquired whether the doctor had come by to which I responded that she hadn't. I am sure that she must have been concerned, but she never expressed this. She was very composed and told me not to worry. She came back at the end of her shift and we waited together. This was comforting. We did not say much. We just waited.

Around 6:00 p.m., Dr. Donovan finally returned. I was scared to receive the news but I had to know. She spoke to Leah and me togeth-er. She apologized for not returning at noon as she promised and she told us that the surgery turned out to be a long and very difficult oper-ation. Oh my God I thought. Is my beloved going to live? She told us that cancer was found deep into the pelvic area and that Yvonne had three primary cancers. I was crushed! My life was being torn apart right in front of my eyes. I was listening intensely as she continued. "Her ovaries, her colon and her uterus were cancerous. A full hysterectomy was performed with removal of the ovaries and a section of the colon. These parts will be sent to the Pathology Lab for further analysis." The doctor said that they believed that they had gotten all the cancer but they couldn't be sure. Yvonne would have chemotherapy later to ensure that all the cancer was eradicated. Leah wanted to know the prognosis and all the doctor would say is that it could be a fight. She told us that Yvonne was in recovery and still unconscious and would be there for a while. She told us that Yvonne was very cold; she had been opened for a long time and had lost a lot of body heat and blood. She would be wrapped in heavy thermal blankets and she would be under a heat lamp and was on a respirator to assist her breathing. We could go and see her later but she would not be coherent and would not recognize us. She answered all our questions and then left.

After the doctor left I cried openly and unashamedly. I was scared, really scared. The reality that Yvonne might not recover had sunk in. Until this time, I had somehow expected that she would survive. She was a fighter and had great faith in God. Now I began to face the possibility that I might lose her. I could not imagine life without her. I needed her. My life would be useless without her. Through it all Leah comforted me. She was strong, not even shedding a tear. I needed her strength to help me through this. Leah held me while she told me that God would give Yvonne life. She told me that Yvonne's strength, her faith, her desire to live would help her survive. Leah excused herself and went to the women's room. There, I later found out, she cried her heart out.

It was fourteen hours later (around 10:00 p.m.), that we were allowed to go to the recovery room and see Yvonne. She was the only patient still in recovery. All others had gone to their respective rooms, but my love was still fighting for her life. Her vital signs were stabilized but she was unrecognizable! My beloved was on a gurney, hooked-up to a respirator, and wrapped in a heavy thermal blanket, with her head covered, and under heat lamps just as the doctor said she would be. Her face was dreadfully swollen and I was exceedingly pained as I saw her lying there, so very still. I whispered to her and told her that I loved her, but she gave no sign that she heard me or even recognized that anyone was there. My heart sank a little deeper and I prayed that she had heard my voice. Leah and I left around 10:30 p.m. Circumstances were not working out as I had anticipated. I was so focused on the events of that day that I could not remember where my children were at the time.

I was blinded by tears as I drove home unaware of what my next moves were going to be. Was Yvonne going to make it through the night? I sped up hoping to get home soon, in case there was a call from the hospital. What was I going to tell the children? I hadn't even spoken with them during the day. I prayed that they were asleep for I was too broken up to speak with them. It was 11:00 p.m. when I arrived home. Robert and my mother-in-law were up. I could sense that my mother-in-law was sad and Rob looked at me with questioning eyes as I entered the kitchen. Rob wanted to talk, but I told him that I would be down as soon as I checked on Danielle. She was asleep and I reached over and kissed her gently not wanting to wake her. Robert knew that things did not go well at the hospital. I was unaware about how much he knew, but he needed to know the truth. He was eighteen years, a young man, and I did not want to hide his mother's condition from him.

We embraced each other when I entered the kitchen and I broke into tears. "Dad, everything is going to be O.K., everything is going to be O.K." I told him about the day's events and the need for all of us to continue praying. Robert looked at me and said: "Dad, do not worry, Mom is going to be all right. I know she is going to be all right." I wanted to believe him but he did not see his mother in the recovery room. He did not hear the doctor's words or touched his mother's cold ashen hand or see her unrecognizable swollen face. I did.

When we came back the following day they had removed Yvonne to the Intensive Care Unit, a move I had not anticipated. This was not going well for me but I knew that she would receive special care that would hasten her recovery. She remained in ICU for some time and I cannot remember the actual length of her stay, but I remember her being unconscious for the duration of the time. Later, we were thrilled when the doctor informed us that Yvonne was being returned to her room. This move told us that she was on the road to recovery. Although she gradually recovered, it took some time before she overcame her grogginess.

I think the next several days were quite difficult for Yvonne. We often prayed with her as she drifted in and out of consciousness. She was being challenged in her faith but she held fast. Her faith never wavered. She never once doubted that she would recover. In fact, she took it for granted. I don't know how she persevered. I thought of a lot of things I had read in the Bible. I thought of how God had allowed Job to be challenged in his beliefs and through it all he never doubted God. I thought of how Jesus had been challenged by Satan in the desert when he fasted for forty days and was told that if he were the Son of God he could make stones into bread. I recalled how Satan had taken Jesus to the mountain top and tempted him to cast himself down to the earth below and how Satan promised him all the earth if Christ would bow down and worship him. Through all of this Jesus avoided temptation and never betrayed his trust in God. Yvonne was a child of God who had learned to trust him during the years. Her faith was strong in a similar manner. She lay there quite ill and she was a source of inspiration for all of us who attended her. She was a silent witness. My faith was growing stronger.

After a day or so, I reluctantly returned to work hoping that I would engross myself in my work, thereby keeping my mind off Yvonne, but my mind was always on her and her well being. I wanted her well and home with us. Every day, I rushed home and then to the hospital. I cannot even remember communicating with the children. I cannot remember their presence, but I knew that they were loved and well taken care of. I stayed overnight with Yvonne in her room, although she was unconscious of my presence. I wanted to be close to her. The nurses on duty were very kind and very helpful. They showed me where their coffee station and refrigerator were and told me to help myself to coffee and juice. I'd known health professionals who were simply working at their jobs to earn money but these were caring people who took the time to treat patients with dignity and were sensitive to their families.

After nine days we had the pleasure of taking Yvonne home where she would continue her recovery. I knew it would not be easy for her, but she was well enough to leave. She had come a long way and the road ahead might be rocky but I was depending on her faith in God to carry her through the rest of the way. Chemotherapy lay ahead, she did not know this and I did not know how she would respond but no matter what, I would always love her and be there for her.

14

Amazing Grace

The bravest sight in the world,
is a man fighting against the odds.
Franklin K. Lane

Operating Room
Date: 5-17-89
Time: 12:20 P.M.
Blood test results (partial):

Tests	Yvonne	Normal / Range.
RBC (Red Blood Count)	3.43 Low	4.20 – 5.40
HGB	10.2 Low	11.5 – 16.0
HCT	26.7 Low	35 – 47
MCV	78 Low	79 – 99
MCH	26.2 Low	27 – 32

Recovery Room – Date: May 17, 1989 – Time: 18:30 p.m.

Vital Signs	Yvonne	Normal / Range
Blood Pressure	80 / 55 Low	120 / 80
Pulse	76 Low	80 / 100
RR (Respiration)	20 Low	20 – 24
Temperature	94.28 Low	98.6
Skin color	Yellow	Pink

Breathing Intubated and spontaneously. Bilaterally clear but diminished. Oxygen 100% Breathing with the aid of an oxygen tank

Notes:
Patient was put under heat shield to increase body temperature.
Anesthesiologist remarks:

Post op anesthetic plan is to let patient breathe via the E.T.T/T-piece until patient warms a bit and regains her strength.

Recovery Room – May 17, 1989

The voice resonated in my head like a distant echo carried by the wind. "Mrs. Williams, Mrs. Williams, can you hear me?" My head felt heavy as if weighted down by a heavy load. I wrestled helplessly to move in response to the unfamiliar voice that was calling my name. As I tried to open my eyelids, they felt weighty as if I had been asleep for an eternity and the muscles had lost their elasticity and were too weak to keep them open. Once again I tried opening them but I could not see. Although vision is the dominant human sense and my sight was temporarily clouded, my hearing was sharp. Under these abnormal circumstances, hearing had become my dominant sense. I heard unrecognizable voices as if in the distance, the humming of machines and someone distinctively asking me if I was cold. The memory of the coldness I experienced then sends shivers throughout my body even today.

"Are you cold, Mrs. Williams?" the soft, pleasant voice asked rhetorically already knowing the answer. I shivered from head to toe in response. A coldness like I had never felt before had taken over my body. It felt as it was being exuded deep from within producing constant shivers. Not even the warm covering that was placed on me eradicated the horrific feeling of being slowly frozen.

I was unaware of my presence, surroundings, or the day's activities, especially my flirtation with death. I was oblivious to the allies around me—the nurses, doctors, family, the respirator that assisted my breathing and the heat tank that hovered over me in hopes of increasing my body temperature from 94.28 to 98.6. I lay helplessly motionless, desperately wanting to communicate. My limbs did not respond to the movement signals my brain was generating. I tried raising my hands, then my legs, but they resisted as if they were pinned down by an invisible weight. I attempted swallowing and realized that there was a foreign object in my throat. It was exclusively mine. It was unrecognizable and I could not share my discomfort with anyone but there was a strong involuntary sensation that I had to rid my throat of it. The feeling was so strong and pronounced that I focused all my energy on determining the best possible way to get rid of it. I remembered I ran my tongue on this impervious object and decided that I could cut through it with my teeth. It was an unconscious psychological and logical survival criterion. It was incredulous! My mind was constantly working although I was unconscious of my state. As my survival gear kicked in, I started to gnaw on the object putting extreme pressure

with my teeth in a saw-like fashion, hoping to cut it in half....
Unconsciousness.

Intensive Care Unit – May 18, 1989
Time: 8:30 p.m.
Temperature: 96.8
RR (Respiration): 20-24
Skin Color: Pink tinge, skin cool but dry
Oxygen: 40% (Transport monitor)

I was now experiencing brief moments of consciousness, but still unable to clearly focus my eyes. I was unaware of my environment, the date, day, or my transferral to ICU the previous night. There was still no recollection of any internal or environmental stimuli or any other bodily sensations, not even the coldness and the brief gnawing of the tube during the recovery process. It seemed as if my other senses were placed on a back burner as my body adjusted to the shock of surgery. I guess time had elapsed, when I heard a man's voice whispering in my ear. His voice was distinct. "You are beautiful, Mrs. Williams, stay with me. Work with me. Yes, Mrs. Williams, work with me. Good, work with me. Great!" I cannot remember his request or in what way my assistance was needed. In some obscure way, these words reinforced my will to continue. On another occasion the voice was recognizable, it was my husband's—William. I was unaware of his presence until I heard him say: "This is your husband, William." I, in turn, whispered in jest, "William who?" Hoping to ignite laughter, but I later learned that William thought that I did not recognize his voice.

15

My Benediction

"I asked God for strength, that I might achieve
I was made weak, that I might learn humbly to obey.
I asked for health, that I might do great things,
I was give infirmity, that I might do better things.
Almost despite myself, my unspoken prayers were answered.
I am, among all men, most richly blessed.
I was given life, that I might enjoy all things.
I got nothing that I asked for—but everything that I hoped for."

Death loosened its tight hold on me allowing me to be transferred from ICU back to my private room on May 19, at 2:15 p.m.

Although I was drowsy from Demerol and Phergan I was being given for pain, I felt the presence of someone hovering over me, the touch to my face was familiar, the kiss on my cheek gentle. Blinking several times I tried to extricate the haze that obliterated my vision, but the person's face was still a blur. The feeling of connectivity between us was strong. My voice hushed, too weak to utter a simple "Hi" or "Hello," but my mind raced with curiosity. Who is it? I know this person! The scent was familiar. The voice was full of love as the person rhetorically whispered in my ear. "Hello, sweetheart, how are you? You are doing fine." Ah, it was Leah....Silence.

I immediately recognized the familiar voice to be that of Dr. Donovan. It seemed as if I was unconsciously and anxiously waiting to hear from her, because her voice sparked a keen alertness, feelings of joy and excitement although I was groggy from the medication and unaware of my surroundings.

"Hello, Yvonne, this is Dr. Donovan. How are you feeling today?" There's no memory of my response but her engagement immediately jogged my consciousness into the realization that my present state was due to surgery, and it was for cancer.

Dr. Donovan asked the visitors to leave save for the immediate family (William, Leah and my mother). There was a brief moment of apprehensive concern as I heard the movement of people leaving. Who are they? Apparently, I must have been asleep when they arrived. Although I was drowsy from the medication, I was bent on hearing what she had to say. The full details of Dr. Donovan's conversation are unclear, but I distinctly remember her stating that she had performed a complete hysterectomy.

"I had to remove both ovaries Yvonne, because they were cancerous." Gently touching my hand as if conveying empathy, she continued. "Yvonne, the cancer in your endometrium was invasive and penetrated deep into the pelvic area."

"I knew it, I knew I had ovarian cancer. God revealed it to me. Everything will be all right. You have done your part and He is doing His," I whispered dazed with Demerol. The room was painfully silent, no one spoke they were fully cognizant of the gravity of my condition....Unconsciousness.

Dr. Kasper's voice was gentle, his touch soft as he woke me, "Mrs. Williams, this is Dr. Kasper. How are you feeling today?"

I felt trance-like as if I was awakened from a drunken stupor. It took a while for me to get my bearing and synergy of thought before responding. My words were slurred and jumbled as I responded.

"Hello, Dr. Kasper."

"Mrs. Williams, the surgery was successful.".... Unconsciousness.

I recognized the distinctive voices of Janet King and Anthony Bartolo, my dear friends. Their laughter filled the room and for an instant, my consciousness joined in....silence.

Ah, Robert's voice! I must have been asleep when he came in. His silhouetted frame moved back and forth as he mingled his talk with laughter. Someone responded, young, a male, but unrecognizable. I wanted to participate and tell him that everything was going to be all right. There were so many questions, so many things I wished to share....silence.

There was much laughter and talking in the room when I awoke. My hearing was sharp: William, Leah, Mom, Bruce and Carol Cutting. Their voices brought much joy....silence.

It was days before the drowsiness of pain medication wore off and my gaining of full consciousness. This awareness was precipitated by horrendous nauseated and tender throat. The crushed ice given to me was soothing to my parched throat but did not cure the sick feeling.

Suddenly, I recollected the earlier experience with the object in my throat. It was no longer there....silence.

How excruciatingly unbearable the pain! I had no idea of the precise locations or the cause, but it seemed as if every part of my body pulsated with it. The urge to cry out in agony was pressing, but I was too weak even to do so. As I lay huddled motionless, with teeth clenched, I thought, when one is in pain, each moment feels like a lifetime. The shot of Demerol I was given by the nurse would soon bring relief....silence.

The rustling noise in the room woke me. I was confused and did not know where I was. It took a while for me to corral my faculties and get my bearings before I opened my eyes. Leah slowly turned as if she was conscious of the eyes that were staring at her back. An awkward smile broke on my face—a smile of recognition. She broke into a responsive smile and moved towards my bed realizing that I had recognized her. Our eyes met and clenched for a second. Her face was the first I recognized. Leaning over, she gently kissed me and I felt the warmth and wetness of her tears as they fell upon my cheeks. Moving in a professional manner, Leah washed and dressed me and changed the linen on my bed in no time. Looking at her with much love, I reached for her hand and held it.

Tenuously I opened my eyes and embraced the early morning sunrise that hovered above the hospital window and imprinted its brilliance on the external red brick wall. For a while, I focused on the imprint as it grew with the rising sun. Suddenly it struck me I was not awakened by the palpitation of intense pain but incredible heartburn. Nevertheless, I was very alert and felt much improved than previous days. There was an unexplained excitement plus I had a cravenous appetite. I did not know if it was caused by my progress or by the beautiful invigorating sunlight that ignited an urge to get up and go outdoors. I wanted to sit up in the yellow colored recliner that was tucked in the corner of the room. I wished to bathe and I wanted to walk.

As my soul rejoiced in the goodness of the Lord, I brought my bed to a sitting position. The attending nurse was delighted to see me awake and sitting up. She offered to assist me in cleaning up but I declined. I wanted to wait for Leah whose arrival was soon.

"Hello, Leah." I said with my singsong Trinidadian voice.

"Hello, my dear."

My sister walked towards my bed and smiled down fondly at me and then tearfully thanked God for His miraculous blessings.

"Leah, I want to sit up in the yellow recliner."

She smiled in agreement and said, "Good."

After her daily routine, she summoned the nurse and they careful-ly assisted me out of bed on to the recliner. Leah tucked pillows around me providing added comfort and support. There was such a feeling of accomplishment, just to sit up. But what an effort! My head was dizzy, my breathing became labored and I felt exhausted. I hardly expected to be so incapacitated and weak. I was more so surprised that I could not move without the assistance of someone. Leah sang softly Mamma's favorite song, "His eyes are on the sparrow and I know He watches me," as she professionally performed her daily duties. I looked at her with candor; she was always on schedule to see me, never complain-ing about doing double duty, never a harsh word and always with a smile. There was overwhelming tenderness towards Leah. What love! How blessed I was. I bowed my head and thanked God.

Saturday afternoon brought many visitors. I saw my Danielle for the first time since surgery and my heart skipped a beat and jumped for joy as she leaned over and kissed me on the cheek, whispering softly, "Mom, I am glad you are O.K." I am sure she had been around but I was unaware of her presence. I noticed that she slowly moved out of the way of the adults as they made me comfortable.

Later that afternoon, I was glad to see my nephews and I smiled as they entered the room. As the younger nephew just six years old entered the room, I heard him say in his distinct Trinidadian voice.

"Daddy, who's dat?"

"Aunt Yvonne," was the response.

Surprised, I listened attentively.

"I mean that?" He inquired with intense quizzicality and pointing towards my bed as if he was misunderstood.

"Aunt Yvonne," was the response.

"It does not look like her, that person looks like a Chinese," he responded naively.

I smiled and asked for a mirror. I wanted to see what he saw. No one had a mirror and although one was attached to the hospital overbed table that was next to my bed, no one made an effort to give it to me. My inquisitiveness was short lived and I did not pursue the need to see the unrecognizable me. I was unaware that the 11 1/2 liters of crystalloid I was given during surgery in order to stabilize my blood pressure and prevent me from having cardiac arrest had artificially inflated my body weight.

The urge to stay in bed was compelling, and as I contemplated on what I should do, I was particularly drawn to the healing of Peter's mother-in-law found in Matthew 8:15: "He touched her hand and the fever left her, and she rose and served him." This gave rise to further reflections of other miracles Jesus performed while on earth. "He then said to the paralytic—Rise, take up your bed and go home." Matthew 9:6, 9:25 "He went in and took her by the hand, and the girl rose." These miracles were reactive. My faith in God was strong, but I was drawn to remember that faith is an action word and "Faith without works is dead." I was willing to take up my bed and walk. My will to live circumvented comfort. As soon as my family arrived, I asked for their assistance in getting up.

"I want to walk. Please help me up." I said breathlessly. I found that talking left me short winded. Asking and receiving the nurse's permission, William put on my slippers and robe then he and Rob gingerly helped me on to my feet while my mother and Danielle kept all the tubes out of the way. I felt like an inactive puppet as I struggled to stand even with the assistance of William and Robert. Let me tell you, it was a harrowing experience. I swayed with dizziness and felt as if I was going to faint. William and Robert's grasp tightened on my arms as they supported my weight. My legs felt rubbery and I had to sit on the bed in order to gain my composure. It was under these circumstances I had to make the decision whether I would trust God and indeed take up my bed and walk.

"Are you sure you are ready to do this?" William inquired, showing concern.

"Yes." Remembering Mamma's teaching: "That one should not stay in bed if one could get up." I was also thinking that, I had to increase my heart rate so that enough oxygen could flow throughout my body. I needed to increase the capacity of my lungs and get my vital organs back in gear. This was tantamount to a timely discharge from the hospital and full recovery. I whispered a prayer under my breath and mentally prepared myself.

William cushioned me with his right arm and Robert with his left. Danielle held the tubes while my mother kept the IV pole from getting in my way. My movements were deliberate as I ambulated out of the room. Each step was methodical and painstakingly slow. This first move was the most difficult and the short walk was a process of stop and go but I persevered. The nurses expressed their pleasure upon seeing me up and they cheered me on as I walked past their station. This show of encouragement pumped up my adrenaline and my will to continue. Inadvertently, the walk had to be cut short because my legs could no longer sustain my weight. I was out of breath and totally exhausted when I returned to my room. Exhausted though I was, I felt satisfied that I had accomplished a milestone. I was on my way.

There was now some familiarity about the room. The cellophaned baskets of fruit, flowers, plants and floral wallpaper brought lightness and hominess to my chancy confinement. Most of my cognitive senses had returned and I was sleeping less. My speech was more coherent and faces were easily recognized. The visits of Drs. Donovan and Kasper were particularly rewarding, as they showed genuine pleasure with my progress.

Although the nurses were aware of my status, I enthusiastically informed each shift of my progress. Still, they responded with surprised interest, excitement and encouragement. In retrospect, the reason I was hospitalized was not foremost in my mind. I never once heard the word cancer mentioned, neither did I think about it. I guess I filed away Dr. Donovan's conversation and the family members didn't bring it up. Probably, I was taken up with immediate events like, pain and heartburn. The cheering section only showed interest in my recuperation and my eagerness to be discharged.

I was now able to get out of bed by myself, but I still needed assistance getting into it. I continued my daily walks, short though they were. This gave me the opportunity to visit with many patients who were hospitalized with similar conditions. Some of them were scared and I was able to offer some comfort.

Since surgery, the pain was neverending and the night of May 22 was no different, every fiber of my body ached painfully. Unable to do anything about my condition but take the prescribed medication, I reached the conclusion that no pain ever lasts forever. In spite of this, I needed relief and decided to seek divine intervention determined to turn my tormentor into teacher. After prayer and contemplation, I realized that pain always accompanies the healing process, whether mental emotional, spiritual or physical. I was definitely going through a healing process. Remembering "As a man thinketh in his heart so is he," I decided to practice the unskilled art of visualization. With eyes closed, I repeated, "Yes God, work the remainder of the cancer cells out of my body, yes, God, work them out." I visualized my body being cleansed from head to toe of all remaining cancer cells, as a full glass being drained. My body relaxed, and all the horrors of pain subsided. After, I termed my pain the healing pain. No longer was I huddled in pain but my body relaxed when I prayed and visualized the healing process. Prayer is really therapeutic and provides psycho spiritual healing. The mind and body are truly one and once again I was lured to realize that the mind is the most powerful tool.

Drs. Donovan and Kasper kept up their steady rounds. But on the morning of May 23rd, Dr. Lieberman showed up instead of Dr.

Donovan. Although a young Resident, she was experienced in bedside manners. I must say, she had a good teacher. What a breath of fresh air she was! Checking my scar, she remarked, "This is healing nicely, the staples have begun to fall out, so I'll remove the rest today." Dr. Lieberman slowly took the staples out, one by one, causing me as little pain as the procedure allowed. The last one was out! Wow! Another milestone, thanks to God.

The staples were out, I was gaining my strength, I was going to have my first bath and my discharge from the hospital was set for the 24th of May. Home sweet home.

Reflective, I took a good look at my person. My feet, hands, fingers and face still swollen. Slowly I ran my fingers through my hair, then along my arms and hands actually touching my body with consciousness. I spent some time genuinely scrutinizing my hands—the looseness of the skin, the whiteness of my palms, the pallor of my fingernails. The pink tinge was gone. For the first time I noticed the intricate lattice work of very fine lines which extended from the back of my hands and increased in size as they ran into my palms forming my unique palm prints. I am alive!

In the past, I was fooled into believing that I had the luxury of time and I often behaved likewise. Now I understood that tomorrow was not guaranteed. In the past I had seen where acquiring great wealth and saving for tomorrow without enjoying some today was the only thrust in the lives of some. I had also seen many die without being able to enjoy their investments or collect on their Social Security. I was forced to recollect a quote from King Solomon, Ecclesiastics 2:24, which states: "There is nothing better for a man that he should eat and drink and find enjoyment in his toil. Sometimes a man who has toiled with wisdom and knowledge and skill must leave all to be enjoyed by a man who did not toil for it. God's gift to man is that every man should eat and drink and take pleasure in his toil."

Leah soon arrived and prepared the essentials necessary for me to take a shower. The sound of water flowing in the bathroom brought excitement. I was walking three times a day and I felt strong. Leah suggested that I take a metal chair to sit on while I showered. I do not need a chair. This was a strange suggestion since I had been exercising. I wanted to stand in the shower and allow the vibration of the warm water to beat against my body.

Leah adhered to my wishes and removed the chair from the bathroom. Well, I was in for the shock of my life! As the warm refreshing water began to beat against my body, it felt as if every bit of strength was simultaneously being drained. I had to hold on to the metal bar for fear of falling. Leah was standing outside the shower probably with a smile on her face waiting to be called.

"Leah, help," I whispered. She immediately reached in and held me. I stood limply desperately holding on to the metal bar with what little strength I had left. Leah helped me out of the shower, limp and helpless like an invalid. She combed my hair and then dressed me. It became quite obvious to me that my recuperative period might be longer than I had anticipated.

As I sat while my sister took care of me, I looked at my frail body and concluded that; illness stirs the soul and brings gentleness and frailness to the body. Humility, dependency, and softness of speech accompany this change. They hold the body captive and puts it into submission. Comparing sickness to old age, Mamma summed it up well: "Once a man, twice a child." I did not understand it then, I understood now.

May 24, 1989

It was May 24, 1989, the day of my discharge from Baystate Medical Center. I awoke early and looked through the window. It was raining. Returning to bed, I used the constant beat of the raindrops against the windowpane to lull me to sleep, but my sleep was constantly interrupted by the excitement of going home. Thoughts of being in familiar surroundings, with the ability to move about unencumbered were welcomed. I was itchy to get dressed, go outdoors, smell the flowers and walk barefooted on the lawn. But most of all I wanted to be with my family and sleep in my own bed.

As I waited for the breaking of dawn. It gave me an opportunity for reflection. I realized that my life is only worth the value I was willing to place on it. Not monetary value, but the quality of being. I was given a second chance, blessed with new beginnings. This, I knew, would be accompanied with new challenges. This new path was unknown and could be arduous, but even for this, I was truly grateful.

Getting out of bed, I drifted to the window, it was still dark outside. Philosophically and retrospectively I thought, in spite of all my heartaches: "I would not exchange the sorrows of my heart for the joys of the multitude. And I would not have the tears that sadness makes flow from my every part turn into laughter. I would that my life remain a tear and a smile. A tear to purify my heart and give me understanding of life's secrets and hidden things. A smile to draw me nigh to the sons of my kind and to be a symbol of my glorification," to my God: Kahill Gibran. I was willing to move forward with singleness of purpose in: "Seeking first the kingdom of God and His righteousness," knowing that "all things will be added."

Looking at my watch, I saw it was only 6:10 a.m., too early to shower and change. Taking my Bible in hand I decided that whatever chapter my finger touched when I opened the Bible, is what I would read (this was a game Leah and I played as children). I opened my Bible and my finger was on Psalms 30. I read:

"I will extol thee, O Lord, for
thou hast drawn me up,
and hast not let my foes rejoice over me.
O Lord my God, I cried to thee for help,
and thou hast healed me.
O Lord, thou has brought up my soul from Sheol,
restored me to life from among
those gone down to the pit.
Sing praises to the Lord, Oh you His saints,
and give thanks to His holy name.
For His anger is but for a moment,
and His favor is for a lifetime.
Weeping may tarry for the night,
but joy comes with the morning.
As for me, I said in my prosperity,
"I shall never be moved."
By thy favor, O Lord,
Thou hast established me as a strong mountain:
Thou didn't hide my face, I was dismayed.
To thee, O Lord, I cried:
and to the Lord I made my supplication:
What profit is there in my death,
if I go down to the pit?
Will the dust praise thee?
Will it tell of thy faithfulness?
Hear, o Lord, and be gracious to me!
Thou hast turned for me my
mourning into dancing;
Thou hast loosed my sackcloth
and girded me with gladness,
That my soul may praise thee and not be silent.
O lord my God, I will give
thanks to thee forever."

This was incredible! How appropriate! This was no coincidence or happenstance. This was my prayer, my answer, my reinforcement of faith, my healing. "God is in this place!" I cried with thanksgiving. I would continue to stand firm in my belief, I would not doubt or lose hope. God is the source of my strength. He would never bring me this far and leave me. God did not promise me a world without pain, but He promised to give me the strength to carry on.

Presumably, I dozed off because it was full daylight when next I looked through the window. The sky was still overcast and the night's thunderous rain had trickled to drizzle. This did not tarnish the excitement of my departure. I sat on the bed hoping that William would arrive earlier than expected. Restless with excitement I looked at the clock for the hundredth time. It was now 7:00 a.m. Good, William should be up. I dialed my home telephone number. It rang several times before a sleepy William answered it.

"Guess what today is?" I asked alert and full of excitement.

"You are coming home, my darling."

"Yes, yes, yes! Please do not be late."

"I will be there soon," he said with excitement.

Not long after, William, Leah and mom walked in the hospital room full of energy and excitement.

With laughter in his voice, William said. "Aren't you ready?"

"No, I was waiting for someone to help me get dressed."

"I will enjoy that," my husband responded with laughter in his voice. Oh, the wonderful sound of laughter.

The room was filled with spontaneous laughter. The nurses came in curious to see what was going on.

"What's going on in here, we do not want to miss out on the fun."

"Join in, I am homeward bound."

"Don't be in such a hurry to leave, your discharge papers are not ready. We are going to miss you around here, Yvonne. You've been an inspiration to us all."

"Thanks for the wonderful care and encouragement. I will be back to visit," I responded my voice light with bliss.

At about 12:20 p.m., all my dismissal papers were completed and the staff nurse carefully reviewed them with William and I.

The nurses said their good-byes with tear-filled eyes and I cried as I departed. Looking at the room, I vowed never to return to this place, but also thinking that. "Parting is such sweet sorrow," I was going to miss the staff. What a raucous parade we must have presented as we caravaned down the hall. An orderly wheeling me, William behind the nurse's aide, followed by Leah carrying my belongings and my mother wheeling a cart full of plants and flowers.

When the automatic doors opened as we exited the hospital, I squinted at the bright glare of daylight. The wind sprinkled with rain softly brushed against my face. The fresh air was exhilarating but an unknown sadness suddenly overtook me.

Mom and Leah transported the plants and flowers in one car and I accompanied William in his. On the way home, William followed the route he took when he visited me avoiding potholes that were carved out by the salt and winter's harsh weather. Although the sites along the route were familiar, for I had seen them numerous times before, I viewed them with renewed interest; there was newness to them—the streets, buildings, homes even the trees.

William turned on to one of the main streets, which was about two miles from home. As we drove pass the cemetery, we simultaneously looked at it, then at each other. We drove in silence, each thinking our own thoughts. I thought: "To everything there is a season, and a time to every purpose under the heaven: A time to be born, and a time to die." It was not my time to die. I had a rare opportunity to live, and live my purpose and I was willing to do whatever it takes to preserve it. Beaming with the thought of new beginnings, I viewed our home in the distance. The flowers were in full bloom, the lawn thick and green, the hedges neatly manicured. It was obvious that my mother was busy; she loved gardening, and was blessed with a green thumb. William reached out and gently squeezed my hands then whispered, "You are home, honey." I was moved to tears but it was short lived as Leah and my mother rushed out the front door when they heard the car engine. They were full of excitement and moved with joviality; my mother clapped her hands stating, "You're home" and Leah was full of smiles and tears. They acted as if they were seeing me for the first time that day. Home, sweet home.

The pleasant spicy aroma of West Indian cooking greeted me as I entered the front door but I was too weak and tired to check out the pots. William assisted me upstairs and I was glad for the support of the bed after climbing the stairs. I thought I would get home, change and take a short walk around the house and breathe the fresh country air, but I was exhausted and wished someone had carried me upstairs instead. It was a matter of the mind willing, but the body was indeed weak.

16

Home Sweet Home

Go home to thy friends,
and tell them how great things
the Lord hath done for thee,
and had compassion on thee.
—Mark 5: 19

The tray of food my mother brought into the bedroom per my request looked appetizing but I was not hungry. I set the tray aside in hopes of eating later.

The vibration of a door slammed shut woke me. I looked at the clock and noticed that it was 3:00 p.m. I had slept for almost two hours and I was unaware of the removal of the tray of food from my bedside.

"Is Mom home?" Not waiting for an answer, the patter of footsteps headed upstairs. Danielle's voice was music to my ears and I swelled with excitement as I anticipated her entrance. She burst into the room.

"Hi, Mom, how are you? I am glad to see you, do you need anything?" She uttered it all without taking a breath or waiting for an answer and with a big grin plastered on her face. Her long, thick hair fell on my face as she reached over and kissed me on the cheek and squeezed my body with her little hands exuberating joy. Danielle lay across the bed and proceeded to fill me on the events at school as if I was never gone. She had kept these details indelibly in her mind, waiting for the appropriate time to share them with me.

I had not given thought to moments like these while hospitalized; now I was glad to be here for her. "Oh, Mom, I just remembered this," she would often interject remembering something about a friend or teacher. I listened attentively as she gesticulated and acted out parts of the occurrences. During the last nine days this young child, my daughter, had willingly taken a back seat without complaining or insisting on her own way. Now it was her time. No one was around and boy, she was making the most of it. I guess I was dozing off because she reached over and pulled the covers over me as she said, "I guess I'll leave now, so you can rest."

Kissing me on the cheeks, she whispered. "I knew you were going to live and come home."

Taken back by her statement, I asked, "Why, sweetheart?"

"The night you told us that you had cancer, you said you were going to live and be with us for a long time. You have always told us the truth." With that, she tiptoed out of the room with a finger on her lips as if not to disturb me. What would have happened if things had not proceeded the way I had anticipated then.

Surprised that my statements had such an impact on her, I was thankful to be alive and I promised to continue on the new path I had taken.

⸺✦⸺

The loud talking and laughing woke me. The house was always alive with activity when Robert was home. I couldn't wait to see his smiling face. Robert walked into the bedroom followed by a section of the posse, Tim, tall, handsome and blonde with grayish blue eyes: Will, good-looking and husky and Kevin, dashing, charming and reserved.

"Hey, Mom, you look great, good to have you home." Robert said, full of energy as he planted a kiss on my forehead.

He was followed by a unison of, "Hi, Mrs. Williams, glad to have you home," from the threesome.

"Hello to all." They, too, had a lot to share. They filled me in on their latest girlfriends and some of their escapades. I knew what they were doing; they were here to cheer me up and their goal was being accomplished. These young men are wonderful, I thought as they left with the same commotion, laughing and loud talking as when they had come in.

Mom came up to see if I was ready to eat, but I was still not hungry.

In a coaxing voice, she said. "Yvonne, you must eat. Just have a little honey."

"Probably I'll have something later," I told her.

"That's what you said four hours ago. Can I prepare something else for you?" she asked, disappointed.

"Well, what about some warm Soya milk?"

Within minutes the Soya milk was brought up, but I only drank a couple mouthfuls and that was a struggle. All I wanted to do was sleep.

It was 8:30 a.m. the next day when I awoke. Turning to get up, I noticed someone next to me, sound asleep. It was Leah. Not wanting to disturb her peaceful sleep, I tried to get out of bed to use the bathroom. Feeling the vibration of the bed, she awoke and assisted me, then she fell right back asleep as if she had not slept for a long while. Leah needed the rest. She had performed double duty for the last two weeks.

The freshly squeezed orange juice and oatmeal with raisins I was served for breakfast did not look appetizing. I drank a little of the orange juice but I found the oatmeal to be tasteless. Unable to complete the meal, I set the tray aside. I knew my appetite would return, but I was not hungry at the moment. After a while, my mother came up to view my progress. Her coercing did not work. The sight of the meal brought on nausea.

"Please, Yvonne, eat a little," Mom urged.

"I'll eat a little later," I promised.

I had a craving for stewed lentil peas, sliced ripe plantains, avocado, codfish with tomatoes and onions, and steamed broccoli. Soon I was presented with my request. I ate a slice of plantain and a little lentil peas but I could not eat anything else. Furthermore, the scent of broccoli repulsed me. Needless to say, Mom was disappointed.

"What can I prepare for you, Yvonne? You need your strength, you must eat a little more." Mom stressed in a concerned voice.

"The broccoli has a funny scent which is upsetting my stomach. I am no longer hungry." I informed her, glad for any excuse not to eat.

Dinnertime produced the same results—no appetite. I drank some juice and feverishly picked over the food. The loss of appetite did not concern me.

Although the country air was fresh and exhilarating I found it extremely difficult walking up and down the stairs to take my daily walk. Instead of walking twice a day, I increased the distance and walked once with the assistance of my mother and the children. The eight-inch scar was healing nicely and the only irritation it presented was a mild itch. The pain lingered but I continued with visualization that helped ease the discomfort. All my teeth were painful and sensitive. Everything had to be at room temperature and reasonably soft for me to eat. This appeared to be another malady, and neither the dentist nor the doctor knew the cause.

Leah continued to do her part by making me comfortable. Every day she systematically propped pillows between my legs, under my arm and behind my back, which brought sweet relief.

I awoke from my afternoon nap to find the tray of untouched food removed. My mother probably took it while I was asleep. That was her usual routine.

"Hello, sis." I was thrilled to see Leah as she entered the bedroom.

"Hi, Yvonne." Leah's greeting was cordial, her behavior standoffish.

I was taken aback. Now what? I knew her well enough to realize that something had to be wrong because she had taken a motherly posture. She came close to my bed and looking me in the eyes, she gesticulated with her index finger, then coolly stated: "You have not been eating for a number of days and this cannot continue. If you do not change now, it will be very difficult down the road. You need nourishment to rebuild your body. We thought that with a change of environment, and home cooking, your appetite would increase, but it hasn't. A glass of orange juice a day is not going to cut it, Yvonne. We are thankful to God for His blessings in bringing you this far. I admire your strength, faith and perseverance and the way you have handled your illness. I do not know if I would have been able to handle three cancers the way you have, but you must eat." So that's it. Mom has been filling her in on the daily happenings. "I don't have to tell you that God helps those who help themselves. You know that. But He is not going to come down and put food in your mouth. If you do not eat, you will die." Walking out the room, Leah closed the door behind her leaving me with her final words: "If you do not eat, you will die."

Her final statement was hard to digest, but it hit me right between the eyes and jolted me into reality. Probably this was the main reason for my prolonged weakness. I believed that with time my appetite would increase, but once again Leah was right. Slowly getting out of bed, I walked to the bathroom into the shower. As the water beat against my frail body, I cried relentlessly. Surprisingly, I realized that in my current condition, I only had a tenuous hold on life and had to eat in order to take a stronghold. Oh, how I wanted to live. Forced to take extraordinary steps, I decided that I would begin eating right away. I was neither angry with Leah nor my mother because I knew the background for what might seem to be a cruel statement. In correcting us, Mamma always said, "Sometimes you have to be cruel to be kind. Sometimes the truth must be told straight instead of being whitewashed." I was grateful for the truth. If I did not eat, I was surely going to die.

There were several ingredients to good health: a balanced diet, adequate water, positive thoughts, exercise, fresh air, sunshine and laughter. I had rationalized my lack of appetite; it takes time to recover, I kept telling myself. To me, I was not emaciated from the weight loss. But my loved ones were looking at my situation in a different light. They saw me slowly deteriorating, losing weight and not getting stronger. The process was the same as the will to live. No one could force or will me to eat. Pressured by my desire to live, it was my decision. Once again I had to take control and make a lifesaving decision.

In tears, I reinforced my determination to live. Proper food is life-giving and life-sustaining, and I had to keep this in front of me. I acknowledged that eating a balanced diet was my immediate goal. This would be a challenge for me, but I could not ignore Philippians 4:13. "I could do all things through Christ which strengthens me." I needed a new infusion of strength.

In implementing my plan to eat, I made a list of my favorite foods and gave it to my mother. I asked her to prepare them for me in small servings. I was faced with the same challenge at dinnertime—no appetite, but my attitude was different towards eating. I forced myself to eat a little but stopped when the nauseated feeling came on. Two hours later, I asked for another small serving that took me two hours to eat. It was a small discomfort in exchange for life.

The morning of May 27, 1989, was an idyllic spring day. Our alarm clocks rang, the doves cooed and the other birds sang in response to daybreak. William often wished the doves would leave their nests in the large pine tree that overshadows our front yard. Although the night's sleep was restless, I couldn't wait to get out of bed and enjoy the glorious day. My mother was thrilled when I told her of my decision to increase the distance of my daily walk. It was easy for her to get caught up by my enthusiasm. "That's good news," she said as she clapped her hands. To her, this was a definite sign of recovery. Dressed in walking clothes, we set out for the walk after having a glass of fruit juice and with my commitment that I would eat upon our return.

"Yvonne, you should have a little more in your stomach before you walk," my mother anxiously insisted.

"The walk will generate an appetite, I'll eat when I return," I said, calming her anxiety.

As I exited the front door, I squinted as the rising sun greeted me with its bright glare. My body was further energized with the flow of adrenaline by the thought of venturing off the beaten path I had slowly trod since my arrival from the hospital. What an euphoric feeling! The dazzle of spring was in the air. The flowers and shrubs that donned the well-manicured yards saluted me in full splendor as I slowly walked. I was thankful for their magnificent tribute. The bouquets of pink and purple rhododendrons hung lightly on their sturdy shrubs while the multicolored tulips, lilacs and gladiolas commanded respect as they adorned the green lawns. The yellow forsythias painted their own pictures while the soft azalea flowers, orange, purple, pink, white and red warmed my heart. Enthralled with this newfound beauty I was unaware of the distance I had covered.

"Do you want to walk further?" Mom asked bringing me back to earth.

I was surprisingly pleased that we had walked about a quarter of a mile and I was not tired, still wanting to savor this renewed appreciation.

I responded with, "This is great! I will let you know when I am tired." Although I was feeling fine, I failed to realize that I had to walk the same distance back and should not wait until I was tired before returning home.

"Don't overdo it the first time," my mother said, with concern in her voice.

After walking for approximately another quarter mile, I noticed my breathing was deeper, my heart rate had increased, my hands were red and slightly swollen and my skin itched. Looking at the redness of my hands—signifying increased blood circulation, I realized that the exercise had increased my heart rate delivering increased oxygen and blood to different parts of my body. Thrilled, I was determined to keep this up on a daily basis. I was aware that exercise not only prolonged life, but also lubricates the inside and increases the body's functionality.

All of a sudden, without warning, tiredness hit me over the head like a sledgehammer deliberately slowing my steps.

"Are you O.K.?"

"Yes."

My mother looked at me with subtle disbelief as she noticed the dramatic change in my pace. She placed her arms around my waist, and assisted me by allowing me to shift my weight on to her. Fortunately for me, she was able to withstand my weight. Each step was slow and calculated as if I was walking in mid-air. As I continued, I prayed, asking God to give me the strength to continue. Finally the house was in sight, my adrenaline kicked in and miraculously, I was able to continue on my own.

The following morning, it took the whole morning for me to drink a glass of juice, eat a few slices of mango and one slice of toast but I did it! My mother celebrated by clapping her hands and thanking God. "Oh, thank you, God," she said as she looked up to the heavens with jubilation. I just smiled and also thanked God.

There were many visitors on May 29th, including Jan, one of my good friends. I wanted a quiet moment to tell her about my illness but the room was crowded.

"Jan, I need to speak with you," I whispered in her ear

"O.K., just tell me when," she said with a smile, as if knowing.

I regretted not telling her before. She had always been one of my major supporters. We loved each other dearly but I had not confided in her. I had indiscriminately reduced my supportive circle and burdened Leah emotionally. Leah did not feel this way, but in retrospect there were others who were willing to share my burdens. Cancer makes you ashamed and secretive because of its close association with death. It unwillingly throws you onto center stage with others looking on. And you have to put up a curtain, only allowing certain persons backstage. I should have been more inclusive with my backstage audience.

17

The Fear of Chemotherapy

I shall not die but live, and declare the works of the Lord.
Psalms 118:17

I felt listless the morning of June 2, 1989, as I sat demurely on the edge of the bed, indecisive about whether to get up or not. Lulled by the warmth of the bed, I found a comfortable position and decided to rest a while, postponing my morning walk. I must have dozed off because the ringing of the telephone startled me into consciousness. Answering it, I was enthused to hear Dr. Donovan's pleasant voice on the other end.

"Good morning, Yvonne, how are you?" She inquired.

There were vast improvements during the last several days and I excitedly informed her of the details; my appetite had improved, I had gained a pound and my endurance had increased, allowing me to walk a half mile without being exhausted. She listened attentively and occasionally interjected with, "That's great, I am glad to hear of your progress."

"Yvonne," Dr. Donovan's voice took on a professional note, "I am pleased to inform you that the pathology report showed that there was no cancer in the Uterus after it was dissected and tested."

"Thank God," I interjected.

"No cancer cells were found in the fluid that was taken from your abdomen. Nor was cancer found in the fat that was removed from the surface of your abdomen."

"That's good news, thank you," I responded, bursting into smiles. I shouted, "God is at work! I knew it!"

"Having three cancers at the same time is very unique," she continued, "so based on the uniqueness and complexity of your case, it was presented at the combined Tumor Board at Baystate Medical

Center on May 30, 1989. It is felt that the best prognosis, in view of the study presented at the ASCO (American Society for Clinical Oncology) meeting by the GOG (Gynecological and Obstetrics Group, Philadelphia, Pennsylvania), it is recommend that you should have follow-up chemotherapy. Six treatments of Carboplatin and Cytoxan afford the best potential cure. At the completion of the treatment, there might be the possibility of going in and have a second look."

In shocked silence, the moments seemed to remain suspended in mid-air.

"Yvonne, do you understand?" the doctor questioned, breaking the heavy silence.

"Yes, I understand." I responded, taken aback.

"Do you have any questions?"

"No, I do not have any questions," I answered in unstable tones.

"Please call the office and set up an appointment as soon as possible, so we can discuss this in detail because I would like to start treatment within a week or so."

"I will. Thank you, good-bye."

The call sent shivers throughout my body. What! Chemotherapy! I sat on the edge of the bed, emotionally frazzled, my eyes transfixed with fright. I was keenly aware of some of the side effects of chemotherapy. No, not chemotherapy anything but that! I shook my head in disbelief, unable to digest the doctor's recommendations. A week was too soon. This was too aggressive for me. Dr. Donovan's statements were stinging, and the thought of taking chemotherapy caustically frightening. My heart palpitated loudly, reverberating within my chest. I had never envisioned participating in chemotherapy. Who does? The liabilities are tremendous and the side effects are sometimes disastrous.

I winced, as the tornado of thoughts and questions riveted my head with imbalance. Why combined therapies of surgery and chemotherapy? What was chemotherapy? Why not radiation? What was the difference between the two? How was it administered? I was scared of both and did not want to experience either. What was the selectivity process? What was the feasibility of me not having it? Chemotherapy treatments do not eradicate cancer else people would not die from the disease. I had heard that it kills both cancerous and non-cancerous cells and sometimes the cancerous cells could build up immunity to the treatments. The immune system has to be strong to fight cancer. Would chemotherapy treatments be subtle and pervasive in breaking down the immune system? I was standing on the threshold of a decision I was faced with and did not want to entertain, but had already accepted.

When it comes to accepting the recommendation to take chemotherapy treatments, the subject is usually spoken in hushed tones with quiet pain. There are no presuppositions, no definitive results, or planned backup. The process is reactionary: there are documented side effects of Carboplatin and Cytoxan, the chemotherapy treatment I was going to receive. But no one would know what my side effects and tolerance would be until the end of the first or second treatment. For only then would the cumulative results be known.

It was not the hair or weight loss, nausea or other side effects that frightened me. My memory was jaded by history and I could not look at chemotherapy treatments objectively. I mentally revisited the times that I was exposed to persons who had experienced these treatments and, to my knowledge, none survived. Focusing my thoughts on them, fear became prominent and I felt emotionally boxed in. My body had not fully recovered from the shock of surgery and I did not know if it was functioning well enough to excrete chemotherapy toxins and recover in time for monthly treatments.

I was flying high with my progress, but as soon as I received the news, the wind was immediately taken out of my sail that had catapulted me. My odyssey seemed neverending and my emotions were once again being trifled with. How could this challenge be a teacher? Right away, though, I had to positively gear my mind up for this new undertaking. My Lord, how I needed a new infusion of strength. I wished that I could accept devastating messages devoid of emotional reactions. But I hasten to remember that even "Jesus wept" at hearing of the death of His friend, Lazarus.

Strewn in doubt, it took the pouring of my soul to God, before I could think clearly. I will trust God to help me through this. God is the source of my being. Although still fearful of the process, my doubts were reconciled and I decided to move ahead with true grit.

The family accepted the news fairly well except for Danielle. She looked at me startled, her eyes wide with concern.

"Mom, would you get very sick and would your hair fall out?" she asked with sadness.

I was shocked by her knowledge of some of the side effects of chemotherapy. Placing my arms around her shoulders, I cuddled her, hoping to erase her fears.

"I do not know, honey," I replied. "What do you know about chemotherapy?" I asked with curiosity.

"While you were in the hospital I saw a movie on TV about a lady who had cancer and she got very sick and lost all her hair when she took chemotherapy."

I was surprised that this twelve-year-old would sit and look at such a grownup movie by herself.

"Why did you look at the movie, Danielle?"

"Because you had cancer and I wanted to know more about it."

"Was anyone with you when you looked at the movie?" I asked surprised and touched.

"No, I wanted to see it alone."

Oh, how I wished I could have been there with her. She probably saw the movie while I was hospitalized. She should have told her father that she saw it. He could have helped calm her fears. I marveled at the strength and tenacity of my twelve-year-old-daughter.

June 6, 1989, the day of Robert's graduation, arrived and I was caught up with excitement. In fact, I moved around with such ease and swiftness that no one would have believed that my body was recuperating from major surgery. I beamed with pride as I looked at my son dressed in his cap and gown. Life is definitely worth living! In five years, it would be Danielle's turn and I planned on being there.

Under the surface of calmness, the following days found me constantly harangued by the thoughts of chemotherapy. There were no cancellation calls as I had hoped for. Therefore, I was left with the stark realization that chemotherapy treatments were inevitable. Nervousness replaced fear. The closer I got to the day, the more nervous I became. It seemed as if this last interruption placed me on a permanent junket. Although I was able to harness my positive energy and continue my healing process, it was difficult to decouple chemotherapy from the destruction of life—the killing of red and white blood cells.

The pre-chemotherapy visit was scheduled for June 13th, and the first treatment was scheduled for Friday, June 16, 1989.

My eyes swelled with tears as the team, Dr. Donovan, Barbara, RN, Oncologist , Lynn, RN, and Gail, the office receptionist, greeted me with such warmth and pride when I visited Dr. Donovan's office on June 13th for my pre-chemotherapy treatment. There was an inner feeling of accomplishment and victory. I wanted to stand up and shout, "I made it! I knew everything was going to be successful. Thanks be to God."

Upon completion of a thorough examination, there was no need for words. The smile on Dr. Donovan's face told it all.

"Everything looks great, Yvonne!"

"Thank you. I knew it!"

"I am very pleased with your recovery thus far and, clinically, I can say you are doing very well," Dr. Donovan informed me as she washed her hands.

It was good news. My next encounter was with Barbara, the oncologist nurse. On the surface, I presented a calm demeanor, but my anxiety was rapidly mounting. I was itchy with unanswered questions and could hardly wait for the meeting. This meeting and the book Chemotherapy and You: A Guide to Self-Help During Treatment were most helpful in understanding the treatment of chemotherapy.

Needing to know more about chemotherapy treatment, Barbara defined it to me by quoting from the book. "Chemotherapy is used most often to describe a method of cancer treatment. The term comes from two words that mean 'chemical' and 'treatment.' Chemotherapy often consists of more than one drug."

Most people have had some type of drug therapy for illness during their lives; for example, taking penicillin for an infection. Although chemotherapy was more toxic, I now understood that it was a drug or combinations of drugs. In the past, I had undergone some form of drug therapy; only now; the dosage would be dramatically increased. This knowledge did not help diminish my fear.

"Why do I have to take chemotherapy instead of radiation?"

Barbara was gracious and answered all of my questions.

"Chemotherapy treatment is really dependent on many different factors. Chemotherapy is used to kill any residual cancer cells that might have evaded radiation or surgery. It is often used when there is a possibility that the cancer may have spread and it is usually prescribed to decrease the possibility of a reoccurrence. There are also some cancers that are specifically treated with chemotherapy and not radiation."

"Will I be able to continue my normal activities?"

"Why, yes. Last winter several women came in, received their treatments, then headed for the ski slopes."

"How will the drugs be administered?"

"The Cytoxan and Carboplatinum will be given intravenously."

"Is the administering painful? Will I experience any negative sensations when they are being administered?"

"I don't think so. No one has ever complained about the treatments being painful. Anyhow, you will be given Ativan which will help you relax."

"Where will the treatments be administered?"

"At this hospital. You have a choice. You can have the treatment administered overnight and spend the night here, or you can have it done during the day then go home after the procedure."

"I will stay overnight." I was thinking that if anything went wrong, I would be in the right place.

"Good, I'll make a note of that and reserve a room for you."

"How often will the treatment be administered?"

"Once a month. Blood work will be performed on you every month prior to your treatment. This will determine if the treatments should continue.

The answers were acceptable and I felt a slight sense of relief, but they did not allay my fears. How can one remove visual memories when similar associations appear? I needed supernatural help, help from God. I was given the necessary requisitions to have my blood work performed that day including a CA-125 and a CEA. The results of my blood work would determine my ability to take chemotherapy treatments.

The results looked comparatively good, so Friday was a go. I left the office, the book Chemotherapy and You hidden under my arm, not wanting anyone to know that I was about to take chemotherapy.

18

Chemotherapy Treatments

O Lord, I cried to thee for help,
and thou hast healed me.
                    —Psalms 30:2

June 16, 1989, the day I dreaded, arrived and I was still unprepared. I had tried ignoring the engagement with crass simplism but it dangled slowly in front of me like a pendulum marking time to the day. Leah was fully aware of my fear. I had confided in her. Therefore she agreed to accompany me and stay during the whole procedure.

Scared, I prayed. "Dear God, my strength is in you but I am fearful of chemotherapy and its side effects. Please Lord, calm my fears and take me successfully through this first treatment."

With cold feet, I checked in for the overnight stay at the hospital on June 16th and was sent to Chapin Wing. It was the same area where I had recuperated from cancer surgery. Walking briskly to the floor, chemotherapy was no longer foremost in my mind, replaced by the thought of seeing those familiar faces and the need to show them how well I was doing. As I entered the ward, the greetings from the nurses were warm as they questioned Leah and me about our visit.

"Hi, Yvonne, how are you?"

"Hi, Leah, back again?"

"Hi, Yvonne, you look great!"

"I am feeling the way I look," was my proud response.

"What are you doing here?"

"I am here for my first chemotherapy treatment," I said, lowering my voice so that the non-medical personnel who were located in the area would not hear my response.

"It is not that bad," was one of the nurse's response sensing my uncertainty.

One of the nurses admitted me to the ward at 9:00 a.m. and the usual admittance protocol was followed. Shortly, Barbara, the oncologist nurse from Dr. Donovan's office, walked into the room. What a pleasant surprise! I never thought of asking who was going to administer the chemotherapy. I took it for granted that since I was going to be hospitalized, one of the nurses or the doctor on duty would perform the procedure.

Taking one look at my arms, Barbara said, "There are no veins, babe." I was given an Ativan pill for relaxation. To help my veins surface, I took a hot bath, then my arms were wrapped in hot towels. After a while a nurse appeared, inserted a needle in the back of my hand and started a saline drip solution. The process of hydration had to be accomplished prior to the treatment. Later, a shot of Carboplatin was given via the IV, then shortly after the Cytoxan was started. Leah sat holding my hand and praying. As the chemotherapy flowed through my veins, and not knowing what to expect, I whispered to Leah.

"I am scared. I do not know what to expect."

"Sssh, everything will be all right. You are in God's hands," she comforted.

It was not that I distrusted God. I had seen the side effects of this treacherous treatment and the memories were hard to shake off.

The morning after, I was awakened with horrendous nausea and a strong urge to regurgitate. I rushed to the sink, located in the room and vomited a couple of times. The expectorant left a bitter taste in my mouth. Mamma used to compare all bitterness to gall. "Yvonne," she would say, "This mauby (a West Indian drink made from the bark of a tree) is as bitter as gall." I had not tasted gall, but this must be what gall tasted like. Walking to the room where beverages were kept, I poured myself a glass of cranberry juice and took a couple packs of crackers in hopes that the combination would settle my stomach. This treatment was not that bad, except for the vomiting and nausea.

I was now ready to go home. I called William and woke him from a deep sleep.

"Hi honey, I am dressed and ready to leave."

"You are?" he exclaimed, surprised that I was up and alert. "How was it?"

"I slept through everything. I cannot remember a thing except when the procedure was first initiated."

"Great! Thanks be to God," he said, relieved, not knowing what to expect.

"When are you going to pick me up?" I asked, anxious to go home.

"I will be there as soon as I can," he responded, lighthearted.

William arrived soon and I was on my way home. One down, and five more to go. Upon my arrival home, I broke into smiles as I entered our bedroom. My mother and Leah had made adjustments to accommodate many of the listed side effects; but for the one I was now experiencing, there was no preparation. A strange, crawly irritability had taken over my body. I felt as if something was crawling through my veins and under my skin. Leah gave me a body rub but the feeling did not go away. I lay in bed, twisting, turning and rubbing my body but the crawly sensation hung on. There were no antidotes and I had to resign myself to this wretched affliction. The warm afternoon breeze made its way through the windows, gently massaging my body and calming my spirit. Unable to do anything about my condition, I prayed and was comforted by the notion that this temporary phenomenon soon would pass.

Leah looked at me with empathy and said, "You must drink a glass of water on the hour as long as you are awake. You have to wash the toxins and the dead cells from your body. I know that you know—just reminding you, love."

"Thanks, I have already started."

I knew that water was vital in the elimination of impurities from the body. It also keeps the kidney and other organs free from toxins and aids in rebuilding cells.

The irritability and crawly feeling lasted for two days. The third day brought sweet relief. I continued eating a well-balanced diet made up of fresh fruits, vegetables, grain and legumes. This was crucial in boosting my immune system. I also was cognizant that the life-giving molecules from foods are killed at certain temperatures. Therefore my rule of thumb was: 70-80% of my daily nutritional intake was fruits and vegetables and at least 10-30% of them were eaten raw.

It was now three days after my first chemotherapy and I was feeling fairly well. In fact, I felt much better than I had expected. I had to keep in mind that it was only the first treatment and I could not gauge the other treatments by the first. I was scheduled to see Dr. Robert J. Kasper on June 19th. I was excited to visit him because my colon was now back in full commission without any apparent problems. Dr. Kasper was elated to see the progress I had made.

The next fourteen days brought bouts of listlessness and fatigue. I had to force myself to get up and not allow the feelings to interfere with my daily activities. There weren't any other obvious side effects and the fear of chemotherapy was slowly being eradicated with the first treatment.

My scheduled monthly visit with Dr. Donovan was July 12, in

preparation for the next bout of chemotherapy due on July 14. I was proceeding extremely well and my weight was on the upswing. The routine visit with Dr. Donovan went well and my blood test results supported a second treatment of chemotherapy that was scheduled for July 14th.

Leah once again accompanied me to the hospital and the same rigorous protocol was followed. As was expected, I slept through the whole procedure and was again awakened by horrendous nausea and the need to regurgitate. The same ghastly bitter aftertaste followed after regurgitation. I followed the same procedure and drank cranberry juice and ate saltine crackers in order to settle my stomach.

Surprisingly, I did not experience the crawly sensation as with the initial treatment. I was indeed thankful to God for that. I kept up my routine and drank a glass of water on the hour for two days and then reverted to eight glasses a day. My progress continued; I was gaining weight, I was now walking two miles a day and I was up and about, performing light duties around the house. Thrilled with my healing and positive outlook, I looked forward to a long, healthy future.

William commented about the pink hue that had returned to my skin. He paid particular attention to my palms as he rubbed them. "I remember the coldness of your hands and pallor of your skin when you were hospitalized," The next surprise was hot flashes. They came on with a vengeance and instinctively I recognized the cause—premature menopause. Both ovaries had been removed during surgery and this was one of the side effects. Is this what I had to look forward to? An internal heat that exuded beads of perspiration, soaking my clothes, was immediately followed by a brief sick feeling. During this period, I did not want to be touched, and the sheets were thrown off, hoping to bring relief. After a short while, my body's internal cooling system was switched on, producing relief and the need to cover up. The experience was bothersome, repetitive and systematically timed.

It was a delight and a blessing, treating my body like a temple. I ate a well-balanced diet. I concentrated on the things that were good and of good report. I trusted God explicitly for everything and worried about nothing. What peace I experienced! Although hair and weight losses were two of the many side effects, my hair grew back and I gained weight. This was indeed a miracle! I was feeling and looking well. I now engaged life and my life force energy was evident.

Excitement was built into my monthly visits with the doctors. The staff showed their exuberance when they saw me and I beamed with satisfaction. I took special interest in finding out all the details of my test results because I knew that they would continue improving. I celebrated the results, especially CEA and CA-125 results.

On August 8th, I saw Dr. Donovan. The examination went well and once again she was pleased with my progress and gave me the O.K. to proceed with the customary blood tests and chemotherapy treatment based on the test results.

I was called on August 9th, and informed by Barbara that my white blood count was low and that the scheduled chemotherapy treatment had to be tentatively postponed until August 18th. A repeat of the tests would be performed on August 16th and if my blood count had improved, then chemotherapy would be performed. I was not one bit fazed by this bit of news, remembering that some things have to cease for a while in order to start up again. God was in charge and I honestly believed that it was not His will for me to have the August 10th treatment. In addition, I believed I was being granted extra time in order for my body to recuperate.

Due to the continued bone marrow depletion and slow white cell recovery, the Cytoxan dosage was reduced from 800 mg to 600 mg, but the Carboplatinum dosage remained unchanged at 575 mg. Chemotherapy treatment proceeded as scheduled on August 18th. There were no significant side effects except for increased tiredness that slowed down my daily activities. With things fairly back to normal, I considered returning to work on a limited basis the beginning of September.

I believed that I was totally free of cancer and it was time to share my experiences with friends and loved ones. Many were shocked and exclaimed:

"But you don't look like you had cancer!"

I am cancer-free, thanks to the doctors and God's intervention," I responded with confidence.

My monthly visit with Dr. Donovan went well as documented in her notes on September 11, 1989:

"The patient is asymptomatic (showing or causing no symptoms). She tolerated her chemotherapy well. Usually vomiting only once on the day after administration of chemotherapy. The patient's blood counts are holding up well.

"The patient's exam today of lymph nodes, breasts, abdomen and pelvis reveal no nodularity (the normal number of cells adaptable to its environment) or masses to suggest tumors. A Pap smear was obtained from the vagina.

"The patient is scheduled to come in for her next course of chemotherapy on Friday if her blood counts today are adequate."

Barbara's call on September 11th was expected but the news that Cytoxan would be dropped from my chemotherapy regimen because of myelosuppression (bone marrow suppression) was unexpected but welcomed. I was O.K. with the decision because I knew that God was carrying me in the palms of his hands and I believed without question that only three treatments of Cytoxan were needed, not six as was previous recommended.

The fourth treatment took place as planned on September 15th. Although the Cytoxan was eliminated, I still experienced the nauseated feeling the morning after. Still disciplined, I kept up the same regimen, eating well and drinking a glass of water on the hour for three months of chemotherapy. But the month of September I slacked off. I was working and back into the swing of things and was not diligently drinking a glass of water on the hour. I was drinking eight glasses of water a day and I thought that was reasonably sufficient. I was feeling fine and my hair was growing, so I figured there wasn't really a need to continue the rigid regimen.

Around the 17th of September, six days after my fourth treatment, heartburn, nausea, vomiting and suppressed appetite were the four infirmities that forcibly took hold of me and pressured me to stop work. I do not know if the lack of voluminous water was the catalyst for these side effects, but whatever the cause, I was now terribly ill and had to cut my return to work short.

Nausea and vomiting was now my routine, instead of drinking water and running to the bathroom. At times I felt too sick even to drink water or get out of bed and I wished that I had stayed on my regimen until the completion of the six treatments. The previous struggles I had with eating were foremost in my mind so I forced myself to eat small portions of food although they refused to stay down. It appeared as if I was losing headway fast as I lay in my bed, sick as a dog. After three torturous days I felt a little better but I was now faced with damage control; eating and getting back on a healthy routine. I continued to force myself to eat and drink water no matter how I felt and, after a few days, I felt much better and I was back to my old self.

With September behind me, I was glad to see Dr. Donovan on the 11th of October in anticipation of my fifth treatment. I was anxious to have the final last two treatments over and done with.

"You are progressing nicely, Yvonne," she informed me.

"God is taking care of me," I said smiling.

"Keep on doing whatever you are doing because it is working.

Probably, I need to go to church. I haven't been recently," she said with a smile. "If your blood results are adequate, we will proceed with your fifth treatment." She responded smiling as she washed her hands.

The test results were adequate and chemotherapy was scheduled for October 14th. This time, I experienced three days of nausea instead of the brief moment after the treatment. But it was not as serious as September's bout. I was now disposed to weakness, which was a side effect of chemotherapy, but I did not allow this to deter my daily walks. In spite of nausea and weakness, I kept up my daily walking ritual but slowed down the pace and decreased the distance.

Dr. Powell, the office Chief, filled in for Dr. Donovan in her absence on November 6, 1989. I had seen him around, busily attending to others, but this was my first encounter with him. Dr. Powell, with his deep southern accent and wonderful smile, was fully apprised of my medical history and had been following it closely. He seemed genuinely pleased and proud of my progress. After the visit, my last course of treatment was tentatively scheduled for November 10th, based on my November 6th blood test results. Great! This was my last month of chemotherapy. I was elated. Oh how I wanted it to be all over.

The assault on my white cells and bone marrow continued, dropping my white cells to a low 2.5 on November 6th. "We will have to wait a while before the next treatment can be performed," Barbara informed me, her voice sounding comforting. I took a genteel position and was not disturbed by the news.

Vitron, an oral iron supplement, was prescribed to combat anemia. Chemotherapy treatments would proceed, provided the results of the November 15th blood tests improved. Barbara called on the afternoon of November 15, 1999. In spite of the supplement, my white cells were still suppressed and my WBC was now 2.3. I was scheduled to have another set of blood tests taken on November 22nd. "If the count is good, we will proceed," Barbara told me, consolingly. The journey was tiresome and I wanted it to end. But in spite of everything I was going through, my faith in God did not waver; neither did my worry meter kick in. I knew without a doubt that God was in control of my situation.

Yet the effects of the suppressed white cells and bone marrow depletion were taking their toll on me, as I was disposed to weakness and found myself needing additional bed rest. In spite of this, I diligently kept up my walking routine, refusing to be engulfed by my bed and the side effects of chemo. Barbara called me with the news on the 23rd; my WBC had dropped to a new low of 2.1.

"Yvonne, in light of this, Dr. Dovonan has recommended that we suspend this last treatment. She would like to see you in her office on December 3rd. More importantly, she wants you to call the office so a CAT scan can be scheduled.

"Why a CAT scan?"

"The doctor will have a baseline by which to monitor your progress."

Thanking her, I hung up the phone. I touched my chest with my fist and repeated with belief, "My God is in charge, and only five treatments of chemotherapy were necessary. Not six." No one could ever convince me otherwise. "Great, great!" I hollered with excitement as I danced around the bedroom with renewed strength and filled with joy. "Thanks be to God!" Finally, finally it was all over. The chemotherapy that I dreaded so much was all over. I picked up the telephone and nervously dialed Leah's number. Uncontrollable tears began to flow.

"Hello, Hello."

"Hello, Leah, this is Yvonne."

"Yvonne, is something wrong?"

"It's over, Leah." Choked up, my voice was reduced to a whisper.

"What's all over?"

"Chemotherapy is all over. Praise be to God."

"Thank God. Who told you?"

"Barbara."

"Fill me in."

As I delved into the conversation with Leah, my belief was reinforced that only five treatments were necessary. There are no setbacks or disappointments when God is in charge. I breathed a deep sigh of relief. Now that the rough part of my journey was over, it was important that I keep my eyes on my goal and not lose focus. It was easy to fall into old patterns, and old habits could easily creep upon me. I was determined not to let this happen.

19

Hallelujah! Hallelujah!

Thou hast turned for me my
Mourning into dancing;
Oh, Lord, my God;
I will give thanks to thee forever more
                                    Psalms 30:10

On December 1st, 1989, my well of tears flowed easy and incessantly. Sad and happy, my emotions were mixed. I wanted to get away
from it all—blood taking, the reminder of chemotherapy, hospital and
hospital beds, the sight of suffering and scents of illness. A change of
scenery was needed. With sadness, I thought of those who had been
on this perilous journey before me and who were still struggling to survive. Oh how my heart bled for them. Unless you have walked in our
shoes you'll never understand the desperate fight. I wanted to say to
them, "Let's take a break from your journey and visit the Caribbean."
But unless your cancer is in remission or you are healed, there are no
breaks. The journey becomes harder, the fight more intense. There is
no rest for the weary.

My December visit to Dr. Donovan was memorable. I knew I was
healed of all cancer and I was electrified with excitement. The routine
examination went smoothly.

"Yvonne," Dr. Donovan said. "I have decided to discontinue your
chemotherapy treatment and not administer the last one. Because of
your history and your inability to continue the treatment, we would like
to perform surgery in order to take a second look."

I was surprised, but not concerned. God was still in charge, and if He
wanted Dr. Donovan to take a second look, then it was O.K. with me.

"I am planning on visiting Trinidad the beginning of December, so
surgery would have to take place upon my return." I informed her.

"That's O.K. with me, Yvonne, there's no rush. I will see you upon your return, and at that time, I will review your status."

That was important to hear. I knew without a doubt that a second-look surgery would not be performed. When God heals, there is no taking back. The family discussed my proposed trip. William and my mother agreed to stay home with Danielle, since Robert was away at Boston College, and Leah agreed to accompany me to Trinidad.

My heart yearned for home. I wanted to see my younger sister, Charlene, Dave, my father, and stepmother, Uncle Godfrey, Patsy, my stepsister, my friends, Agnes, Trevor, Henrietta, Anthony and their children. I hungered for Agnes' sweet bread and pealau, a spicy mixture of meat, pigeon peas and rice. Reminiscing of times past, the singsong voices of my people and laughter danced in my head. A smile engulfed my face as I envisioned walking around the Port of Spain savannah and taking the periodic stops to drink coconut water. My mouth watered with the thought of eating mango, roti and Aunt Una's calaloo, soup made of dasheen leaves, okra, coconut milk and lots of seasonings, sometimes it contains crab meat or lobster. A smile engulfed my face as I remembered the men whistling and teasing their women folks while they tantalizingly walked as if there were no bones in their hips. I longed for Trinidad. There, the atmosphere would provide rest for the weary. I was tired.

--- ◄►► ---

Diego Martin, Trinidad, December 19, 1989

The crisp, cool morning breeze woke me as it brushed against my body as if purposefully caressing it. I looked around the room. The curtains were pressed against the metal bars that protected the open windows. They seemed to be pinned as the soft breeze blew incessantly against them. Leah was sound asleep next to me, and no movements could be heard in the house. Trevor, Agnes and Jason were probably sound asleep. We had been up late liming (hanging around) and ole talking (light conversations about past, current and future happenings) with family and friends. The calypso music in the distance was soft and mellow. Dogs were barking as if in response to each other and the roosters were vocal about their presence. I could not buffer the sounds, so I tiptoed out of bed and strolled to the front porch. Goldie, the dog, barked and wagged her tail with excitement when she saw me, and I am sure, hoping that I would feed her.

I sat on one of the porch chairs but jerked forward from the coldness of the metal. The air was fresh and crisp, but I was immune to its coolness. I looked at the towering green mountains that hovered over the Diego Martin valley. They blocked the sun's full view, but its rays projected over the horizon. As I stared at the trees, they seemed as if they were uniformly planted, making a thick covering for the ground, and a haven for wild animals. My vacation in Trinidad was at its end, just another day. How nostalgic to be back home! Solemn about my soon departure, I wished it could continue for at least another week. The distraction was miraculous!

My visit to Trinidad was in celebration of my total healing. My physical, mental, spiritual and emotional bodies, were now realigned and in harmony, and my connectivity with the Creator was renewed and strengthened. I knew without a doubt that I was victorious over cancer and there would be no need for a second look. God does not give something and then take it away. I was feeling great, and being home in this relaxed atmosphere was climactic to a traumatic journey.

Tears flowed down my cheeks with thankfulness as I sat enjoying the beauty that surrounded me. The experience with cancer had been cataclysmic. Nothing could mar this near tragic lesson that humbled and molded me into a new person. Old attitudes and behaviors had passed away.

In retrospect, the visit to Trinidad could have been my final good-bye. But out of calamity came renewal. Out of dissatisfaction came peace. Out of fear came joy. Out of doubt came strength. Out of pain came joy. Out of long-suffering came healing. Out of despair came courage. Out of distress came a second chance. It was not my final good-bye, thanks to Mamma's and Daddy's early teachings and my willingness to trust God for everything. If it were not for their strong spiritual compass that guided me, I would have lost hope during the trying times. Solomon's wisdom was carried forth when he wrote "Train up a child in the way he/she should grow, and when he/she gets old he/she would not depart from it." The journey was made easier and the challenges conquerable because I believed without a doubt that God's word would not change.

The distraction of Trinidad was necessary, but it was now time to return to America, to William and the children. I was missing them.

I saw Dr. Donovan on December 27th, 1989, with the belief that there would be no second look. Her letter on December said it all.

Date: 12-27-89
NAME: YVONNE WILLIAMS

The patient is status post TAH-BSO, ometectomy, bowel resection for a combination of endometrial cancer, ovarian and colon cancer. The patient received five courses of chemotherapy and this had to be stopped because of persistent neutropenia. The patient does have a history of sarcoidosis and her white count has been stabilized at approximately 2,000. The patient feels well and is doing well. Her CT-scan is negative. Her CA-125 is negative. Her CEA is negative. In view of her negative results and inability to continue with adjutant therapy we do not recommend a second look surgery.

The patient's exam is normal. The lungs are clear. Her breasts are benign without any mass or nodularity. Her abdomen is soft, non-tender, without any masses or organomegaly. There is no adenopathy, no peripheral edema. On pelvic exam the perineum is normal and the vagina is clear. Bimanual exam is negative.

The impression is the patient clinically is free of disease. We will plan to see the patient back in two months, at which time we will recheck her blood counts, her CA-125 and her CEA and will start monitoring her every three months following that visit.
Julia T. Donovan, M.D.
cc: Dr. Baez and Dr. Kasper

No second look! I was not just clinically free of cancer, I was a victor over disease and free of the behaviors that causes cancer.

Unable to break the galling yoke I had placed on my life, my body had cried out for change in order to save my life. I had answered its agonizing cry by the renewing of my mind and my behavior. I was indeed a new creature looking towards the future with a thirst for living.

Through this traumatic experience, I am convinced that nothing happens without reason. Things do not manifest themselves without cause, and there are no chance meetings. But through it all, my belief that there is a God, a God who is faithful had been reinforced.

From my experience I know it is very difficult to hold on to hope in the face of death. But let me assure you there are no risks in explicitly trusting God for your life, in helping you to get over the hump. Without faith in this God, I would be dead. The battle was too much for me to engage alone. Each person, though, is responsible for his or her body. We are our own caretakers and our primary caregivers. We must not and cannot depend on anyone else or anything to take care of our bodies.

What a difficult lesson for me! What a traumatic experience! But through it all, through it all, I took my brick walls, laid them flat; and made them stepping stones.

—Yvonne L. Williams

Updates

May 17, 2000, I celebrated eleven years of victory over cancer with no recurrence!

William and I are still very much in love and enjoying all of God's blessings. After my experience, he has developed a personal relationship with God.

Robert graduated from Boston College in May 1993, and married a classmate, Gail Harris, August 14 of that year. On August 3, 1998, they presented the family with a beautiful baby boy, Kasen Jeffrey Williams. Robert has turned out be a fine son, husband and father.

Danielle has developed into a wonderful secure young lady. On May 17, 1998, we celebrated her graduation from the College of William and Mary. She is currently enrolled in law school.

Mom never returned to Trinidad.

My beloved Leah died October 25, 1992. The loss is tremendous! The void is unfilled. If only I had known then about the ravages of prolonged negative stress I would have been able to help my sister and probably, she would have been here today. But God knows best.

Closing Remarks by Danielle L. Williams

Dear Reader:

My mother has asked me to write the closing remarks of this book. I asked her what exactly did she expect me to say. Her words were, "I don't know, but you will think of something."

Well, I suppose I should begin by telling you a little bit about my mother. As you have already ascertained, she is my mother. Having lived with her all my life, I guess I know her fairly well. My mother is an extremely dedicated person: dedicated to herself, friends, family and, most importantly, to God. She has been a very important person in my life, as well as in the lives many others. You only have to meet my mother once to remember her. Hundreds of shopkeepers all over the world can attest to that. With her keen wit, easy smile, and open heart, it's easy to see why.

I think my mother has always been a giving and positive person. Before her experience with cancer, I can never remember a time when she put herself first. Family, friends, work, the sick and needy, church; these took precedence in my mother's life. Cancer made her realize that her life is a special gift, which she must treat as such. I am truly glad that she learned that lesson. In my heart, I know that my life and the lives of many others would have been drastically different if it were not for my mother. I have often imagined how life would have been if my mother were not with me. It truly scared me.

I hope you enjoyed this book. I hope her story has made you realize (as it has made me) how valuable your life is, how important it is to not give up, to live life to the fullest—and most importantly, to be happy. Today, I am happy to say that I have a family made stronger by my mother's struggle. Through her we have realized how important life and family is. Her strength has fortified our faith in God and each other.

Well, I think you understand my point. My mother is my heroine, and I am glad she is who she is. Remember the phrase my mother coined: "Take your brick walls. Lay them flat, and make them stepping stones."

Sincerely,
Danielle L. Williams